THE
PARANOID'S
Pocket Guide to Mental Disorders
You Can Just Feel Coming On

D0912778

This is a work of humor. The disorders and the information about them are real,
but some facts may have been omitted because the author's debilitating fixation on
his own inadequacy precluded his writing them all down. This is not to be used as
a medical text.

Published by Bloomsbury USA, New York
Distributed to the trade by Holtzbrinck Publishers

All papers used by Bloomsbury USA are natural, recyclable products made from
wood grown in well-managed forests. The manufacturing processes conform to
the environmental regulations of the country of origin.

Cataloging-in-Publication Data is available from the Library of Congress.

ISBN 1-59691-270-7
ISBN-13 978-1-59691-270-0

First U.S. Edition 2007

10 9 8 7 6 5 4 3 2 1

Printed in China by Legend Color Ltd.

THE
PARANOID'S
Pocket Guide to Mental Disorders
You Can Just Feel Coming On

DENNIS DICLAUDIO

BLOOMSBURY

INTRODUCTION

I feel it's necessary to begin *The Paranoid's Pocket Guide to Mental Disorders You Can Just Feel Coming On* with an admission.

Prior to authoring this book, I wrote another book: *The Hypochondriac's Pocket Guide to Horrible Diseases You Probably Already Have*, intended as a humorous guide to some of the more unsettling diseases to which mankind is susceptible. And—because I'm kind of a jerk—I tweaked it so that it would draw out and tease the hypochondriacal tendencies that so many of us carry.

But here's my admission: I'm not a hypochondriac. In fact, if anything, I'm the opposite of a hypochondriac. (A *hyper*chondriac? What is a chondriac, anyway?) I never believe that I'm sick. I could be paralyzed from the eyebrows down and I'd still be fending off friends' attempts to drag me to a hospital. So I'll confess to feeling a small amount of guilt for having written a book designed to make people squirm, particularly when I, myself, was immune to such squirming.

However, karma has a way of setting things right.

I decided that a natural follow-up to a book on physical disorders would be a book on mental disorders. Seemed like an obvious choice.

But then I had to write it. And that's where my miscalculation became apparent.

Here's another admission: I may not be a hypochondriac, but I *am* a world-class neurotic. And not the cute "Oh, you're so wacky" kind of neurotic. The "I can't deal with your neuroses anymore; I'm leaving" kind of neurotic. I may always believe myself to be healthy *physically*, but mentally, I'm a hopeless, blathering, soggy wreck. I must have diagnosed myself with at least 25 percent of the disorders in this book (for the record, Adult Baby Syndrome—page 162—was not one of them), as well as countless others that didn't make the final cut. The fact, alone, that I subjected myself to several months of research into mental disorders that I felt on the cusp of acquiring bespeaks some sort of unhealthy masochistic tendencies.

Thus, karma has its way.

Having a rather intimate understanding of the inner workings of a disordered mind, I thought it might be useful to add a feature to the entries of this book: The Inner Monologue. Each monologue is a narration of the disorder itself. This is an attempt to divorce the mental disorder from the mind it's affecting—imagine the disorder portrayed as one of those little cartoon devils that sits on its victim's shoulder and twists his or her view of the world.

As in the previous book, every disorder recounted here—whether neurological or psychological in nature—is completely real, researched and explained to the best of my ability. And at great personal discomfort on my part.

I hope that you enjoy reading this book as much as I did not enjoy researching it.

—*Dennis J. DiClaudio, Jr., B.A.*

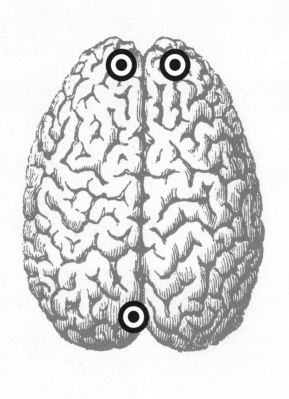

ANXIETY
DISORDERS

Because life's too short to not

spend it worrying.

CEREBROPATHY
(ALSO BRAIN FAG, BRAIN FATIGUE)

Because there's only so much information your brain can handle before it just snaps.

- O Do you sometimes feel intellectually overtaxed?
- O Do you suffer from anxiety or nausea when called upon to think?
- O Are you absolutely certain you answered these questions correctly?

INNER MONOLOGUE

You have to concentrate. Focus on this equation in front of you. You've been at this for hours. Days. But if you just concentrate hard enough you'll get it. It can't be that complicated:

$$S = -\frac{T_0}{2} \int d^2\xi \sqrt{-\det \gamma} \gamma^{\alpha\beta} \partial_\alpha X^\mu \partial_\beta X_\mu$$

Well, T stands for *string tension*. That's easy enough. An ∂_α is the target manifold. What the hell is a target manifold? Who made this nonsense up? This can't mean anything in real life. They're trying to get to you. They made up this ridiculous equation with a bunch of squiggly lines just to make you squirm. But it won't work. You'll show them. You'll show them all.

They're watching you through the walls. They're watching through the book. They want to drive you mad. Well, would a madman take off all his clothes, slather himself down with cream cheese, and streak across campus, loudly professing his sanity? That'll show them.

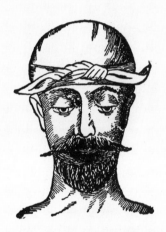

DIAGNOSIS

Cerebropathy, often called Brian Fag, occurs when you push your intellectual energies to their absolute limit. Imagine a gauge inside your head with the needle wavering nervously in the red zone. Your brain reaches a point at which it can't rev any harder, so that the slightest additional input causes the gears to snap violently. Following this "snap," it becomes difficult to remember even simple details. Concentration on anything becomes nearly impossible. Your brain simply feels exhausted. Cerebropathy may also lead to an inability to sleep, extreme anxiety, depression, and possibly full-on dementia.

CAUSALITY

The disorder has been linked to severe mental stress resulting from intellectual over-stimulation and lack of sleep. It may also be caused by an overexposure to other people. It has been known to occur among Japanese office workers, who will sometimes spend more than 80 hours a week at their desks, as well as in West African students struggling to adjust to a Western educational system.

> "Concentration on anything becomes nearly impossible. Your brain simply feels exhausted."

Probably the simplest way to treat Cerebropathy is simply to remove yourself from the stressful situation in which you've landed. If you haven't returned to normal in a few weeks, you may want to seek professional treatment, most likely consisting of psychotherapy and possibly anti-anxiety medication, such as lorazepam.

Of Note . . .

While classic Cerebropathy is considered to be a psychological disorder, the name is sometimes used to describe Encephalopathy, a neurological disorder caused by any number of physical problems, such as liver disease, kidney disease, or a shortage of oxygen to the brain. The symptoms can be virtually identical; however, if left untreated, Encephalopathy may lead to coma and possibly death. So if you find yourself with a case of Cerebropathy, just remember to calm down, and try to relax—otherwise you'll die.

HYPEREXPLEXIA

(ALSO EXAGGERATED STARTLE REACTION,
STIFF-MAN SYNDROME, KOK)

Because everything, everywhere, is always shocking.

QUIZ YOURSELF

○ Are you easily startled?
○ Do loud noises cause you to recoil more than they should?
○ Do your muscles ever clench so tightly you become all but paralyzed?
○ What was that noise?

INNER MONOLOGUE

Good idea bringing her to Count Dracula's Bloody Hell-house of Horrors and Freakatorium for your first date. This is a good change of venue from that French bistro place; that hasn't always worked out so well. There was that one incident when you brought that cute redhead from the video store and the couple at the next table ordered champagne. Waiters should warn you before they pop those bottles open. Jeez, you really freaked out the redhead. Too bad she didn't let you pay her dry cleaning bill.

And there was the time you were walking back from *les toilettes* and the *maitre d'* brushed past you unexpectedly. That caused a scene. You'd think nobody'd ever seen a man freeze solid and fall sideways into a cart full of *soufflé au Grand Marnier* before.

And then there was the time you discovered what *escargots* are. I mean, come on, they should really mention that somewhere on the menu.

Anyway. Count Dracula's Bloody Hellhouse of Horrors and Freakatorium should be a blast.

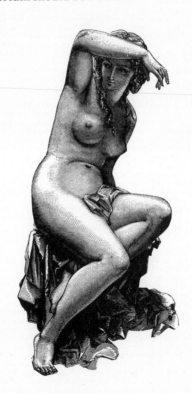

DIAGNOSIS

A sudden loud noise, someone jumping out at you, a polar bear falling through the ceiling and into your living room—all of these things are likely to startle you. And you'll react, as well you should. Your muscles contract, your blood pressure shoots up, you scream, "Ah! A polar bear!" These are all very natural responses to unexpected and irregular stimuli.

But what if your reaction to unexpected and irregular stimuli was a little more . . . exaggerated? What if every time a door slammed shut, you jumped into the air and jerked your limbs wildly? What if every time a salesman at the clothing store appeared from behind a rack of coats to wish you happy shopping, you screamed bloody murder? What if every time your wife reached out to lovingly touch your shoulder, you froze stiff as a board and tipped over like a falling redwood?

That would be Hyperexplexia. And for people who suffer from it, even the smallest of shocks, the lightest of touches will cause an incredibly overblown reaction. In rare cases, the stimulus will cause your muscles to clench up so tightly that you can't move. You can't balance yourself. And then comes slightest breeze and . . . *timber!*

Hyperexplexia is a genetic neurological condition (unlike Hypergraphia (page 96), which is psychological). Which means that when you hear a door slam, even your DNA gets scared.

> "Even the smallest of shocks, the lightest of touches will cause an incredibly overblown reaction."

There is no cure for Hyperexplexia. However, anti-anxiety and anti-spastic medications may be prescribed to make the symptoms more tolerable. And you should probably avoid places like Count Dracula's Bloody Hellhouse of Horrors and Freakatorium.

HYPERSCRUPULOSITY
(ALSO EXCESSIVE RESPONSIBILITY, RESPONSIBILITY OBSESSIVE-COMPULSIVE DISORDER)

Because if only you'd been paying closer attention, everything bad that's ever happened to anyone you know could have been prevented.

QUIZ YOURSELF

- O Do you care about other people?
- O Do you feel responsible when things go poorly?
- O Do you spend a lot of time worrying and fretting about people you love?
- O Do you need to tap your pencil on the table exactly 458 times to keep an asteroid from landing on your sister?

INNER MONOLOGUE

It's your fault. You know that, don't you? Your fault. You should have known. You should have made it your business to know. You should have been paying attention to the traffic reports in Tucson. The wind patterns. You should have flown out to Arizona and examined the brakes on his car. You should have taken a class in automobile repair and kept close tabs on all aspects of the steering mechanism. You should have locked him in his home that day and fed him through the mail slot.

If you had done that, he would still be alive right now. But he's not. He's dead. And it's your fault. This is blood you'll have to carry on your hands for the rest of your life. That guy, whatever his name is, who you met that one time at that party is dead, and it's all your fault. Murderer!

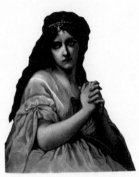

DIAGNOSIS

As you sit comfortably reading this book, a phenomenal number of terrible things are happening in this world. Buses are overturning. Airplanes are crashing. People are falling through poorly constructed sidewalk gratings. Man-eating radioactive tigers are exploding in kindergarten classrooms. Television executives are discussing the new fall season. If you could get a bird's-eye view of civilization, you would be appalled.

And what are you doing, reading? Relaxing? While all of that turpitude is turpituding? For shame! How dare you sit there enjoying yourself when you could be *worrying*. Brooding. Ruminating! With all of this horror happening right now, somebody should take some responsibility. Somebody needs to take some responsibility. Why not *you*?

Welcome to the world of Hyperscrupulosity. You can pick up your hair shirt by the door, and the self-flagellation whips are being waxed at the moment but they'll be ready by noon. From now on, everything bad that happens in the world will be *your fault*. When a friend is hurt in a car accident, you'll know that *you* could have prevented it if only you'd warned him not to drive to pick up milk. When a family member is diagnosed with cancer, you'll know that *you* could have held back the disease if only you'd been more diligent in thinking positive thoughts. When your wife's kindergarten classroom is consumed in a radioactive tiger explosion, you'll know that *you* could have saved her if only you'd touched the bathroom door handle 72 more times. It's a heavy burden you'll bear, but don't worry. You've got more than enough obsessive guilt in you to meet the challenge. Or to feel guilty about not meeting it, anyway.

CAUSALITY

Medical evidence supports the theory that Hyperscrupulosity, like other forms of Obsessive-Compulsive Disorder, is the result of low serotonin levels (which affect mood), as well as abnormal brain activity in the cingula and frontal lobe (which organizes behaviors and regulates emotions).

TREATMENT

Hyperscrupulosity is one of the most difficult forms of OCD to cure. Because sufferers are so consumed by guilt and what is perceived to be others' fates, they are deeply reluctant to let the disorder go. However, cognitive behavioral therapy can help victims realize they don't have nearly as much control over events as they think. And serotonin reuptake inhibitors—such as fluvoxamine or sertraline—may help to regulate brain activity.

Of Note . . .

Say what you will about Hyperscrupulosity, but a thorough search through the Lexis-Nexis database turns up a startling *zero* results for reports of man-eating radioactive tigers exploding in kindergarten classrooms throughout the world. The Obsessive-Compulsives must be doing something right.

SCRUPULOSITY (ALSO

RELIGIOUS OBSESSIVE-COMPULSIVE DISORDER)

Because God is watching everything you do . . .

- ○ Are you religious?
- ○ Are you *really* religious?
- ○ Shouldn't you dress a little more conservatively?
- ○ Are you definitely going to Hell?

INNER MONOLOGUE

You must remember to keep Jesus in your heart. Please, for the love of everything that is good and holy, keep Jesus in your heart! Do not become distracted. This world is a cesspool of sin and temptation. Satan is waiting around every corner to trip you up. Speaking of which, check out this girl coming around the corner. Can you believe she has the indecency to wear a skirt that small? How disgraceful. That's exactly the kind of thing you should avoid. Look, it barely covers her . . .

Oh no. Were you judging, or merely looking? Check for lust in your heart. Check for lust in your heart! Okay, there doesn't appear to be any lust. Just antipathy. But wait—antipathy is not a Christian virtue. Antipathy is a tool of the Devil! You should fill your heart with love for that misguided young lady with the very short skirt. But not lust.

Look at you. How can you claim to have Christ in your heart when you can't even keep your mind off lust for five seconds? What must Jesus think? What would you think of you if you were Jesus? Hold on, are you actually comparing yourself to Jesus Christ, your Lord and Savior? You're a thousand times worse than that unfortunate girl with the short skirt and the incredibly toned thighs! You'd better get yourself to confession immediately. Never mind that that's where you're coming from. Just turn around and go back. Do you think Jesus worried about being inconvenienced when he was dying on the cross for your horrible, horrible sins?

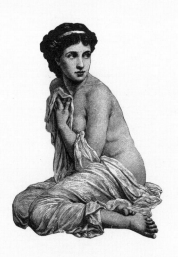

DIAGNOSIS

Scrupulosity is actually a form of Obsessive-Compulsive Disorder, or OCD, in which the obsessive-compulsiveness manifests itself through exceedingly pious behavior. You will find yourself plagued with fears that God is judging you as sinful, that he's watching your every move, just waiting for you to trip up so he can mark your ticket for a bus ride to Hell.

Those with Scrupulosity will find themselves offending Him in any number of ways, including during patently religious actions. Is there a better number of candles you should be burning? Probably. Did you just have an impure thought about the pretty young clerk at the Bible store even though you were trying your best to feel Christ's agony while He was nailed to the cross for *your* sins? You're done for. How will you make it up to Him? Light more candles? Will you have enough? Can you risk another trip to that store?

Scrupulosity is usually considered a problem of Catholics, who excel at guilt, though kosher-conscious Jewish people have been known to give the Catholics a run for their money.

CAUSALITY

Despite conventional wisdom, extreme religious devotion is probably not the cause of most Scrupulosity; rather, the disorder is a manifestation of an obsessive personality. Your brain wants very badly to find something with which to torture you, and if you happen to be religious, that works as well as anything else. Perhaps better. Religion has been used as a mechanism of psychological torture for millennia.

Like other forms of OCD, it is likely caused by an imbalance of serotonin, a neurotransmitter that helps regulate mood, sleep, appetite, and other functions.

TREATMENT

Tendencies of Scrupulosity have been found to respond to certain mood-regulating medications. Also effective is exposure and response prevention therapy, which teaches you to accept the compulsive thoughts as a function of the disorder, understand their cause, and allow them to pass.

No serious religious organization accepts Scrupulosity as a healthy form of religious expression, so most churches, synagogues, ashrams, zendos, and Scientology capsules will offer counseling for it. It's important to remember that at the heart of every major faith is a philosophy of compassion.

Or you could just pray really, really hard and see if God will change His mind about you.

SUSTO (ALSO FRIGHT SICKNESS, ESPANTO, PASMO, TRIPA IDA, PERDIDA DEL ALMA, CHIBIH)

Because you'd lose your soul if it wasn't attached to your body.

QUIZ YOURSELF

○ Do you sometimes feel listless or sad?
○ Do you have trouble maintaining an appetite?
○ Do you suffer from involuntary muscle tics and/or diarrhea?
○ Do you scare easily?
○ It's ten o'clock; do you know where your soul is?

INNER MONOLOGUE

Wh-whoa! That was close. You almost fell right on your face! Those goddamned kids, leaving their toys out in the hallway for somebody to trip over—hold on . . . Where's your soul?

Is it in there? Anywhere? No? Oh, for Pete's sake! You lost your soul again. It's gone. Great, just what you need. You've got those executives coming in from St. Louis for that meeting tomorrow, and now you're going to be sleep-walking through the whole presentation. Muscle tics and trips to the bathroom every five minutes. Marketing's going to be pissed if you don't make a good impression. Of course it's too late to get a *curandero* over here tonight. You can't find a decent shaman healer willing to make house calls anymore anyway.

Damn those kids!

It's always something, isn't it? Toys to trip over in the hallway, strange dogs barking out of nowhere, dead relatives visiting in the middle of the night, and *poof*—your soul just goes!

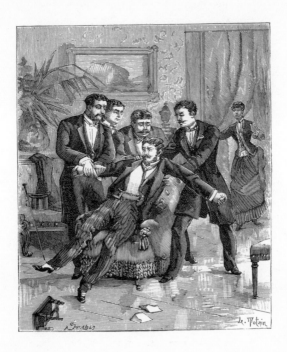

DIAGNOSIS

The good news for people with Susto is that it's unlikely the soul has actually been displaced. The bad news is, maybe it has. A soul is difficult to pin down. Merriam-Webster defines it as "the immaterial essence, animating principle, or actuating cause of an individual life." The online Urban Dictionary defines it as "the Godson of James Brown and princess of Aretha Franklin." Neither definition is helpful in this case.

Ultimately, however, if you believe you once had a soul and now believe it to be gone, that's a problem—and a defining characteristic of Susto.

Studies show that a lack of soul can cause anxiety, loss of appetite, involuntary muscle tics, diarrhea, depression, and insomnia. In severe cases, Susto can even bring about death. If your brain can convince your eyes they can't see, it stands to reason that it can convince your body it's not alive.

CAUSALITY

Seen predominantly in Mexico, Central America, and South America, Susto episodes typically occur following a sudden shock or trauma to the victim. People have lost their souls after waking up and finding themselves in bed with a dead person, but the cause needn't be that extreme; you can lose your soul simply if you fall off a horse, or if a dog barks unexpectedly near you, or if the corner store is out of your favorite flavor of ice cream.

"Ultimately, if you believe you once had a soul and now believe it to be gone, that's a problem."

TREATMENT

Should you experience Susto, you'll want to locate a *curandero* (healer) to administer a *limpia* (cleansing) as soon as possible. The *curandero* will lay you down on a cross of tinfoil, rub your body with herbs, say some prayers, and then jump over you. Your soul should come flying right back, though the steps may need to be repeated a few times if your soul is particularly far away.

If, for some reason, you're unable to find a *curandero*, cognitive behavioral therapy under the care of a licensed psychologist may also prove effective.

TAIJIN KYOFUSHO
(ALSO ANTHROPHOBIA)

Because something you do could embarrass somebody else, and that would be the worst thing in the world.

QUIZ YOURSELF

○ Do you ever worry that you might be making someone else's life intolerable with your body odor?

○ Do you worry that someone will be wildly offended if you look them in the eye?

○ Do you fear the possibility that you'll blush, and therefore make somebody else blush?

INNER MONOLOGUE

Subways are the worst. The absolute worst. All these people packed into this little metal box. You should have taken a cab. It's so hot, and it's been hours since you last showered. You must smell terrible. This poor lady you're pressed up against—hopefully she can't smell how rank you are. What a terrible predicament for her. And she seems like such a pleasant—

Oh my God! She looked at you. She looked right at you. *In the eye.* That must be so terribly awkward for her, to have accidentally locked her glance with yours. She must be devastated. Whatever you do, don't blush—you might embarrass her because she embarrassed you! That would be so embarrassing! She would be devastated. She'd be devastated that you're devastated that she's devastated. That would be devastating.

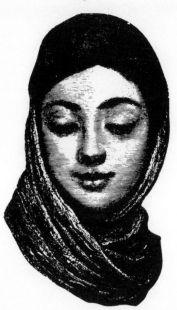

DIAGNOSIS

At first glance, *Taijin Kyofusho* may seem similar to a number of common social phobias. Broken into four categories,

Taijin Kyofusho is a fear of blushing (a symptom of Social Anxiety Disorder), a fear of having a deformed body (Body Dysmorphic Disorder—see page 194), a fear of making eye contact (similar to many anxiety symptoms), and a fear of one's own body odor (Olfactory Reference Syndrome). So why does this collection of disorders exist as its own disorder? And why does it have such an exotic-sounding name? Here's why:

Taijin Kyofusho is generally considered a Japanese culture-specific disorder. The distinction here is that the sufferer fears not simply having these problems and being judged harshly because of them, but rather offending or embarrassing other people with them. Politeness is paramount in Japanese culture.

People with *Taijin Kyofusho* basically walk around in mortal fear of embarrassing others. As you might imagine, this can be socially crippling, especially in a country as populated as Japan, where there are at least ten or fifteen potential embarrassees around every corner.

CAUSALITY

Exact causes are unknown, but research points to a convergence of certain sociological and neurological forces (public transportation ridership possibly among them).

By Western standards, the symptoms of *Taijin Kyofusho* would most likely be treated through cognitive behavioral therapy, in which the patient is taught to work through his or her fears, locate the root of them, and gradually replace them with more positive thoughts. Or they'd be given drugs. Westerners like prescribing drugs. In this case, Prozac might be appropriate.

A Japanese doctor would be more likely to prescribe Morita Therapy, a treatment based on the principles of Zen Buddhism involving mandatory bed rest, diary writing, physical labor, and discussions of positive thinking. Through this, the patient is taught not to lose his or her anxieties, but to accept them for what they are, present but unable to govern his or her life. Eventually, the patient learns to remain constructive despite his or her emotions and to lead a purpose-oriented lifestyle.

Of Note . . .

Morita Therapy has been embraced by some Western psychologists, and it has proven somewhat successful for curing social anxiety and shyness; on the other hand, you could say that about a lot of things.

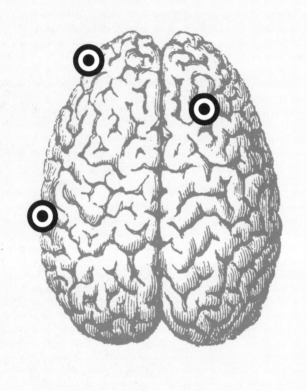

DISSOCIATIVE
DISORDERS

Because things are not always as pleasant
as they first appear.

CAPGRAS SYNDROME
(ALSO CAPGRAS DELUSION)

Because for all you know, your mother could secretly be a robot.

QUIZ YOURSELF

- ○ Do you believe somebody close to you has been replaced by an imposter?
- ○ How about by an alien?
- ○ A robot?
- ○ A shape-shifting wizard?
- ○ Can you really tell the difference? Really?

INNER MONOLOGUE

Who does this bastard think he's fooling? Does he really think you wouldn't recognize your own husband? You've been living with him for decades! And then this fraud comes along, sleeps on your husband's side of the bed, wears *his* clothes, goes to *his* job, drinks with *his* old college friends, and leaves the toothpaste cap on top of the toilet for some completely frustrating unknown reason exactly like your husband does, and does he really believe you're suddenly going to think he's your husband? Fat chance!

He does look an awful lot like him, you'll grant him that. . . . Actually, he looks exactly like your husband. And he smells like your husband—that distinctive combo of stale beer and oily hair. Wow, this imposter guy really did his homework. And he talks like your husband, in that same condescending tone like he's explaining something to a four-year-old with a learning disability. Still, you'd know your husband if you saw him. And this isn't him.

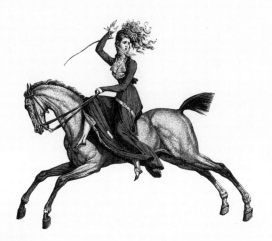

DIAGNOSIS

Actual incidents of people being kidnapped and replaced by identical look-alikes are extremely rare. In fact, it never happens. But for victims of Capgras Syndrome, it seems to happen a little too often. And, frankly, even once is a little too often for that kind of thing.

Should you find yourself coming down with Capgras Syndrome, you might begin to suspect that your spouse is an imposter, someone who looks exactly like your wife or husband but is actually just pretending. Alternately, you might become convinced that your child is an alien shape-shifter just waiting to catch you off guard so it can suck your memory out through your face. Or it could be your dog. Two words for you: "robot dog." Think about it.

In many cases, the victim of Capgras Syndrome may simply accept the imposter's presence. (Who can say why some look-alike, act-alike stranger is willing to cook for you? Does it matter?) Other times, the perceived switch causes considerable problems. (If you're seriously convinced that somebody took your loved one and replaced him or her with an automated diesel-powered Simubot 3000, you might decide to crack open that Simubot with a kitchen knife and pull out its clockwork gears. Simubots can be put back together; husbands and wives, as a rule, cannot.)

CAUSALITY

Capgras Syndrome may be caused by a stroke, drug overdose, blunt trauma to the head, or other event that interferes with emotional exchange mechanisms in the brain. If, following such an event, you see a person for whom you normally feel a strong emotional connection but find those feelings suddenly absent, your brain may scramble to find an explanation. If you look at your wife, whom you love with all your heart, and feel nothing, then it can't be your wife—it must be someone (or something) else.

TREATMENT

In some cases, Capgras Syndrome goes away on its own. The brain establishes new connections, or you decide that you prefer this new robot-wife anyway. Cognitive behavioral therapy, in which a therapist helps you understand the implausibility of your beliefs, can also be effective. Failing this, anti-psychotic drugs, such as Thorazine, or electroconvulsive therapy, in which electrical shocks are applied to the brain to induce a small seizure, may be prescribed.

Of Note . . .

If your brain is really intent on screwing with you, you may decide that your loved one has been replaced not by one imposter, but by *multiple* imposters taking turns—all of them waiting, waiting for their chance to watch *Wheel of Fortune* with you. Devious.

CONFABULATION

*Because the fact that people don't believe you spent the afternoon
deep-sea diving with Jacques Cousteau doesn't mean
you don't clearly remember it happening.*

QUIZ YOURSELF

- O Do you sometimes find yourself forgetting details of the day?
- O Do your recollections of events often differ from others'?
- O Have you ever piloted an atomic-powered spaceship?

INNER MONOLOGUE

When your wife insisted you spent last weekend, cleaning the gutters, you thought she was crazy. Why would she make up something so ridiculous? Obviously you weren't doing anything of the sort. How could you, when you plainly remember spending the past three weeks racing a bicycle across the French countryside in the Tour de France?

Okay, so she made a good argument when she pointed out that you're not exactly in prime physical shape. But that's what made your victory so sweet! The pulling ahead of Lance Armstrong, just meters before the finish line, is a memory you'll cherish forever.

Sure, the hospital report stating you'd been admitted after falling off the roof would have taken some work on your wife's part, but that could've been forged. And the neighbors could have been bribed into testifying they watched you get carted into the ambulance. But the video footage of you holding up last Sunday's newspaper while stating your name and then losing your balance and falling onto your head in the driveway? That's impressive. Why would you have been holding up two forms of government ID to the camera, anyway?

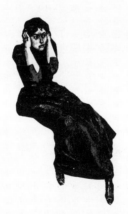

DIAGNOSIS

Confabulation is a memory disorder that's either somewhat scary or kind of cool, depending on how you look at it. If you're the type of person who views the glass as half empty, it might be unnerving to imagine that everything you believe, every memory you have, might be false—an absolute construction of your brain. However, you're the type of person who views the chalice (which was a birthday gift from Poseidon, God of the Sea, in commemoration of your successfully leading a defense of the Kingdom of Atlantis against marauding battalions of evil hammerhead sharks) as half full, you might see the fun in remembering a much more "interesting" reality than most people.

These confabulations are false memories, rather than lies or hallucinations. You don't ever actually see these things, but you believe they actually occurred, even when the facts suggest otherwise. Many confabulations are boring. You might recount eating Frosted Flakes for breakfast, when in fact you had Apple Jacks. That's not the kind of detail that rocks anybody's world, so people probably won't call you on it. However, if you mention that you ate Frosted Flakes with Tony the Tiger himself, you may notice some raised eyebrows.

CAUSALITY

The memory loss inherent in Confabulation is thought to occur due to a rupture of the anterior communicating artery in the brain, as from an aneurism or head injury. This rupture stops the flow of oxygenated blood to the basal forebrain, which handles memory recall, causing a sort of amnesia. If you simultaneously suffer damage to the frontal lobe, which handles self-awareness, you may not realize you've forgotten things. Your brain will grapple to formulate a new memory without your awareness. Often, this is a boring memory, stolen from yesterday's breakfast. Other times, it's something entirely fantastical.

TREATMENT

Through counseling, patients may learn, over the course of months, to separate factual memories from false ones. But they usually will not regain proper memory function.

Of Note . . .

According to one report of Confabulation from the mid-1950s, a young man who had suffered a head injury during a car accident woke up in a hospital room claiming he had been injured in an atomic explosion triggered by a crash-landing of his spaceship. Trusted sources have since indicated, however, that his spaceship landing went very smoothly.

COTARD'S SYNDROME
(ALSO COTARD'S DELUSION, NIHILISTIC
DELUSIONAL DISORDER, NEGATION DELIRIUM)

Because if you were dead, would anybody even tell you?

QUIZ YOURSELF

○ Do you sometimes feel pangs of anxiety?
○ Do you suffer from waves of guilt or depression?
○ Do you find yourself feeling displaced from reality or from your body?
○ Do you sometimes question your own existence?
○ Are you dead?

INNER MONOLOGUE

Here's your family, or what was your family, sitting down before a large Sunday meal. You remember those Sunday meals; you looked forward to them. Did you ever feel quite so alive, so much a part of the world, as you did when you sat down to break bread with the people you loved? A palpable sense of belonging filled the air, mingling with the aroma of lovingly prepared food. And here they continue their weekly tradition, while you, now a malodorous corpse, feel your internal organs slowly fall into decay.

Pay attention—your Uncle Frank is asking if you want the broccoli. But what is broccoli to a man who is no more?

What do the dead care for steamed vegetables? And melted cheese? What kind of cheese is that? Oh, Pepper Jack used to be your favorite. Can you recall those halcyon days when your body was still fresh and vibrant, before your veins were thick with stagnant fluid—blood polluted with the bacteria of putrefaction—when you would slice Pepper Jack cheese into small bits and eat it with Ritz crackers while watching *The Price is Right*? How the days course past!

And your family—these fools—do they not understand the gravity of sitting to dine with a man who has crossed death's threshold? Are they so shameless that they can indulge in a Sunday feast with a cadaver beside them? Why do they not do what must be done and carry your lifeless form outside and put pick to soil, carving out a proper grave? Why do they only want you to pass the mashed potatoes?

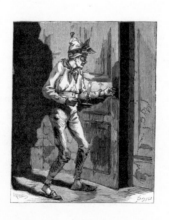

DIAGNOSIS

Cotard's Syndrome is the belief that you are dead, or that you don't exist, or that your body has dissipated into the universe and is no longer sentient. Or, possibly, that you never existed in the first place. If you're thinking it doesn't make sense that a person could believe *anything* if they weren't around to believe it, you're absolutely correct. It doesn't make sense. But if you don't exist, what do you know? You're hardly a reliable source.

If suffering from Cotard's Syndrome, you might feel a complete disconnect between yourself and the world around you. The dining room table beneath your fingers may seem distant, and although you can feel it, you know, deep down, that you do not occupy space as it does. You may feel your skin rotting on your bones, your internal organs liquefying, your body dissolving into the atmosphere. It's not, of course. But nothing anyone says can shake your fervent belief that you are no more, or perhaps never were.

CAUSALITY

Most people with Cotard's Syndrome are also diagnosed as depressive. But then thinking you're dead might be somewhat depressing, so it's hard to know whether one is causing the other, or vice versa.

It's generally believed that the disorder is linked to damage in the brain, in a way very similar to Capgras Syndrome (page 36). In fact, it's hypothesized that Cotard's is a more severe form of Capgras, with the delusional focus directed inwards instead of outwards.

TREATMENT

Cognitive behavioral therapy, antidepressants, and/or anti-psychotic medication may have positive effects, but only in rare cases. Studies have shown electro-convulsive therapy, which redirects blood flow within the brain, to be somewhat more effective.

If none of this works, man, you're dead. *Zing!*

Of Note . . .

Many victims of Cotard's Syndrome also experience delusions of immortality—reason being if you are dead and still eating cheese and watching *The Price is Right*, then in some sense you must have traversed, or beaten, death. And if the most exciting thing you can come up with to do after achieving immortality is sit around watching game shows, then the accompanying depression makes a lot of sense.

DEPERSONALIZATION DISORDER

Because being alive doesn't necessarily mean you have to feel that way.

QUIZ YOURSELF

- O Do you sometimes feel listless?
- O Do you have a sense of detachment from the world around you?
- O Do you ever feel like you're a robot, living your life as you were programmed to?

INNER MONOLOGUE

Making a sandwich, making a sandwich, making a sandwich. Getting the mayonnaise, getting the mayonnaise, getting the mayonnaise. Spreading the mayonnaise, spreading the mayonnaise, spreading the mayonnaise. Cutting the sandwich, cutting the sandwich, cutting the sandwich. Bleeding, bleeding, bleeding. Really bleeding, really bleeding, really bleeding. Spraying blood on the counter, spraying blood on the counter, spraying blood on the counter. Getting woozy, getting woozy, getting woozy.

Man, this is so boring.

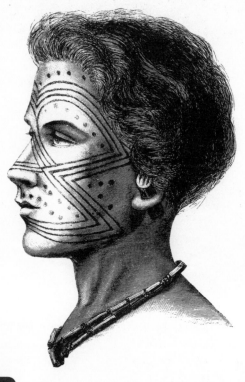

DIAGNOSIS

Depersonalization is an odd little psychological quirk of humanity. It's something that approximately three-quarters of the population experience at one time or another, albeit passingly, often during times of extreme stress. It's those moments when you're looking through your own eyes and seeing the world move around you as though you were

watching someone else's life—a feeling of being discon-
nected. You do things. You go about a daily routine, but
somehow you're not you. Or, you are you, but not the you
you're used to. This will usually last for less than a minute,
and will happen only a handful of times in your life. But
for people who suffer from Depersonalization Disorder, it
is a constant, continual (non)feeling.

The sensation can come on suddenly, and then just never
go away. Sufferers live in perpetual not-quite-numbness/
not-quite-anxiety. It's more like a confusion, sort of. It's
been described as watching your life as if it were a movie.
Or as if you were a robot, or a ghost. Not that you think any
of that's true. That's just what it feels like. You may fear for
your sanity, feel that you've lost your grip on the world. But,
somehow, you manage to live a normal life, in which most
people around you won't even know how you're feeling. You
can imagine how frustrating that could be for you.

CAUSALITY

What causes Depersonalization Disorder? That's not rhe-
torical; that's an actual question. If you know the answer,
please contact every psychological expert right away.

What *is* known is that it is not a neurological problem,
like Cotard's Delusion (page 44), nor a psychotic disorder,

like Schizophrenia. It's almost certainly a psychological problem, along the lines of Panic Disorder or Depressive Disorder. It often occurs after the victim experiences a life-threatening event, such as a car accident or serious illness.

TREATMENT

Depersonalization Disorder will usually dissipate, eventually, without treatment. And even though you *feel* as though you're not connected to reality, you are. Most people just ride it out.

If it doesn't dissipate on its own, psychotherapy has proven helpful. And antipsychotic drugs (though again, it's not a psychotic disorder) and mood stabilizing medications have shown positive effects.

Of Note . . .

The film *Being John Malkovich*—in which a man finds a tunnel that carries him inside the brain of film star John Malkovich—was probably the best representation of Depersonalization Disorder ever put on screen. Not that there have been many attempts. Or any. But the sensation of existing inside another man's head is spot-on.

DISSOCIATIVE FUGUE
(ALSO FUGUE STATE)

Because you never know when you might be lying to yourself about everything in your entire life.

QUIZ YOURSELF

○ Do you sometimes feel confused about your life?
○ Do you ever blank on details from your past?
○ Do you actually believe that you're you?
○ Are you a middle-aged white guy who doesn't speak Spanish picking beans in Colombia?

INNER MONOLOGUE

This is strange. What are you doing in the middle of this field? What are these coffee beans doing in your sack? Why are you picking coffee beans and putting them in a sack? You're a systems analyst. And what's with this hat? Something's not right. Who are these people? Why are they calling you Juan? Your name's not Juan. Is it?

Think. Think. What's going on? What's the last thing you remember? It was morning. Breakfast. You were drinking coffee. You were imagining a simpler, happier life?

Your wife was telling you something. About your brother. Something about her and your brother. She and your brother have been doing something. Together. Wait a minute. Oh, no. Okay, stop thinking! Stop remembering! Just stop now! La la la la la la la la la la la la la la la la la la la la la!!! You are not thinking about this! La la la la la la la la la la la!!! Just pick the damn beans and be happy!

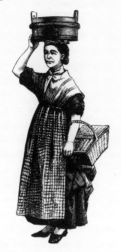

DIAGNOSIS

In layman's terms, Dissociative Fugue is amnesia coupled with running away—often, *far* away. You will lose all memory of your past, then get on a bus and simply go. Once you are someplace sufficiently else, you will create a fresh identity and begin building a new life, possibly a life that you once longed for. For instance, a peaceful coffee bean picker's life instead of a cuckolded husband's.

Diagnosing a person with Dissociative Fugue is next to impossible; he or she will look and act just like anybody else. If you ask about the sufferer's past, you may get some confused stares and mutters, but nothing drastic enough to clue you in. Nor is it possible to recognize when you are suffering from Dissociative Fugue. In the throes of this disorder, you will firmly believe that you are you, even though you are not; you are actually some whole other you.

CAUSALITY

Dissociative Fugue is most often associated with wars, serious injuries, or natural disasters, though the disorder can be triggered by any event so traumatic or stressful that the mind refuses to process it. Instead, the brain shuts down, "wipes the hard drive clean," so to speak, and convinces you to go somewhere you won't be reminded of the situation at hand—in essence, a psychological "do-over."

> "There are few experiences more agonizing than realizing you're not the person you thought you were."

Most cases of Dissociative Fugue will cure themselves on their own. Usually, a victim will discover major inconsistencies in trying to rationalize the past, become very confused, and suddenly snap out of it. Keep in mind, the journey back to reality is often marked by severe depression, grief, shame, and/or suicidal impulses. There are few experiences in life more agonizing than suddenly realizing you're not the person you thought you were and the past several weeks or months of your life have been a fraud . . . not to mention the fact that you now have to return to your former life—the one you couldn't deal with in the first place. Having an emotional support system lined up could prove invaluable.

Of Note . . .

Dissociative Fugue is thought to be somewhat genetic, as many people who suffer from the disorder have family members who have also suffered from it. If your Uncle Charlie once vanished for six months and turned up in Alaska with a tribe of Inuit calling him Amaguq ("father wolf"), be on the lookout. And consider a tattoo of your wife's contact info as a visible reality check.

FREGOLI SYNDROME

Because anyone can be anyone, anywhere, anytime.

QUIZ YOURSELF

○ Are your enemies incredibly well-trained con artists with amazing skills in acting, prosthetics, and illusion?

○ If they were, how would you even know?

INNER MONOLOGUE

He can't still be mad about that bicycle, can he? That was more than twenty years ago. You were just kids. What did you know? But there he is, standing across the street, pretending to be reading the menu in front of that Indian restaurant. He saw you see him, and now he's playing all innocent. He's going inside. Right. Enjoy your Murg Kata Masala, Christopher Welsh. As if . . .

There he is again. He's getting out of a cab—that's a neat trick. How'd he do that? And dressed like a woman now. What fantastic makeup. Wow. He's clearly spent the past few decades training himself in the intricacies of disguise, quick-change, and illusion. And why? All over some stupid three-speed you rolled into the reservoir when you were twelve? Get over it, Chris. This is no way to live your life.

Wait, look. He's going around the corner. He must have figured out you saw through his disguise. Is he gone?

Now, here he comes back around the corner. As a four-year-old boy. Wow. The height alteration alone is astounding. What is he using, mirrors? He's good. You have to admire that. Even if he does kill you over that stupid bike, you have to admire his skill.

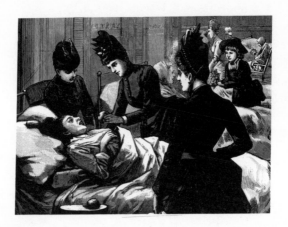

DIAGNOSIS

Fregoli Syndrome is the delusional belief that people you know are either dressing up as random people on the street or are inhabiting their minds—neat tricks, if they were actually happening, which they're not.

People with this disorder will usually fixate on one person from their lives, and will keep seeing that person everywhere. Anyone they see can be that person, even if there isn't the slightest resemblance. But they will *know*, deep in their heart of hearts, that it's the person of their fixation in disguise.

CAUSALITY

Experts are unsure of the exact brain malfunction behind Fregoli Syndrome, but the general belief is that it's caused by a disconnect between cortical areas in the two hemispheres of the brain. Each hemisphere perceives conflicting data, causing the part of your brain that makes sense of things to manufacture explanations for the discrepancy. For instance, if you are receiving one message that says the guy in front of you is a street mime and another saying it's your grandmother, you might rationalize that your grandmother is disguised as a street mime.

This underlying disconnect can be caused by a head injury, stroke, drug overdose, epilepsy, or any of a thousand other things you can do to mess up a brain.

> "You might rationalize that your grandmother is disguised as a street mime."

TREATMENT

Antiepileptic medication, such as carbamazepine, has been shown to have some positive effects, but cognitive behavioral therapy, with its much lower incidence of adverse reactions, is a recommended first step.

Of Note . . .

Fregoli Syndrome is named for twentieth-century Italian actor Leopoldo Fregoli. Fregoli was renowned for his ability to change costumes and assume new identities in mere seconds as his amazed audiences looked on. Audience members suffering from the then-unnamed disorder, however, didn't think he was anything special.

MICROPSIA (ALSO ALICE IN WONDERLAND SYNDROME, LILLIPUT SIGHT, MACROPSIA)

Because size, space, and time are all relative anyway.

QUIZ YOURSELF

- O Do you suffer from feelings of anxiety?
- O Does time ever seem to slip away from you, or crawl to a near stop?
- O Are your hands a different size this morning than they were last night?
- O Does your linoleum floor ever seem like it's made of oatmeal?
- O Which is bigger, your goldfish or your car?

INNER MONOLOGUE

This is troubling . . . your hands weren't always this size, were they? Of course not, otherwise how would they have fit inside your gloves? Or *any* gloves, for that matter? Okay. Calm down. Just sit down and relax. You're not seeing things right. Wait. You *can't* sit—how are you going to fit in that chair? Did somebody replace your furniture with something from a dollhouse?

You need to see somebody, and quickly. Where are the car keys? Shoot! You can't pick them up, they're too big. Plus, they won't fit in the car, let alone the ignition. Just go outside and hail a cab with your massive thumbs. The front door is only a few miles away. If you get a start now, you may be outside by sunup.

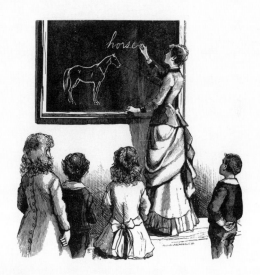

DIAGNOSIS

Victims of Micropsia, or Alice in Wonderland Syndrome, suffer from wild distortions in their perception of reality. Objects seem to lose their God-given size and texture and begin shrinking and growing at random. Even parts of your own body are not immune to the flux. You might look down at your feet and discover they're the size of a side of beef.

Your fingers may grow into long, spindly twigs. Space may also shift. Walking across the room to turn off the TV could seem like a three-day trip. Even time may lose its definitive quality. It could take an hour for the remote control to fall from your tree-branch hand and onto the squishy, spongelike hardwood floor.

It may seem as though physics went on holiday, but you can rest assured that this is not the case. Physics is working diligently, as always; these reality lapses are happening inside your head. Often, they occur in near darkness, when the brain is already taxed due to a lack of spatial reference points.

CAUSALITY

Micropsia is caused by a short circuit in one of the electrical wires inside your brain, in much the same way that a badly wired lamp will flicker. (The metaphor isn't perfect, but it's not as far off as you might imagine.) In many cases, these lapses of perceptive reality are due to epileptic attacks or migraines, both of which are thought to be caused by the faulty firing of nerve cells inside your brain. Doctors don't know precisely why this happens, but theorize it may be caused by a virus or by diet.

> "It may seem as though physics went on holiday, but you can rest assured that this is not the case."

TREATMENT

Unfortunately, unlike with a bad lamp, electrical tape won't be of use. What you may want to do, however, is pay close attention to what you eat: Coffee, chocolate, and red wine have been known to trigger attacks. If you notice a correlation, begin by eliminating the suspected ingredient from your diet. During an episode, your best recourse is to turn on a light, take a few deep breaths, and wait for the worst to subside.

Of Note . . .

The syndrome gets its common name from Lewis Carroll's classic children's book *Alice in Wonderland*. Carroll is known to have suffered from migraines, and it's suspected that much of the bizarre imagery in the book was inspired by the syndrome that would later bear its name.

MIRRORED SELF-MISIDENTIFICATION

Because always there's always that same bastard staring at you every time you go to brush your teeth.

QUIZ YOURSELF

O Do you see the same person over and over at different places throughout the day?

O Do you ever get the feeling you're being watched?

O Do you ever get the feeling you're being stalked?

O Do you ever get the feeling you're being stalked by someone who looks exactly like you and likes to hang out behind your full-length mirror?

INNER MONOLOGUE

There she is again. This is a little much. It's one thing to spy on you from behind storefront displays and the windows of parked cars, but following you into your home—into your bedroom, no less!—to watch you change clothes is definitely going too far. How did she get behind your vanity table anyway? Never mind that. The nerve!

Look at her, so brazenly glowering at you. Like she wants to kill you. That's why she's here, she means to kill you and steal your collection of lighthouse knickknacks. Well, she can't have them. Does she realize how many *years* you've spent collecting them? How many seaside gift shops and antique stores you scoured to find them? As a matter of fact, didn't you see her eyeing the Ziggy commemorative "You light up my life" lighthouse in that antique store? But why pay for her own when she could simply follow you home, kill you, and take yours?

Well, she won't get away with it. She won't. You have to protect yourself, and you have to protect the Ziggy lighthouse.

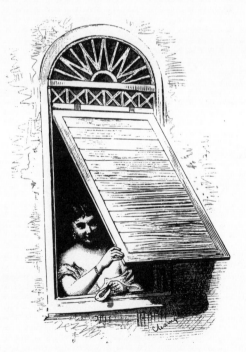

MIRRORED SELF-MISIDENTIFICATION

DIAGNOSIS

You can go anywhere in the world, climb the tallest mountain, dive to the bottom of the deepest sea, wait in line at the slowest DMV, or sit in the audience of the lousiest Broadway musical, but you'll never get away from one particular person: you. Wherever you go, your reflection is certain to follow. Ordinarily, that might not seem so bad—maybe not great, and maybe you don't like being reminded of that increasingly prominent new chin or the deepening lines under your eyes, but it shouldn't be terrifying either. However, for people with Mirrored Self-Misidentification, it can be.

People with the disorder don't recognize their reflection as such. If afflicted, you will think your reflection is somebody else. It might be somebody who bears a striking resemblance to you, but it's not you—rather, it's somebody who loves to follow you around. And if you find that same interloper staring at you every time you look in the mirror, things may get violent.

Mirrored Self-Misidentification is believed to be caused by a defect in the brain that prevents you from connecting a sense of identity or emotional attachment to the image of your face. This defect can be caused by a number of things, including infection, drug overdose, a stroke, or a particularly severe head injury.

"If afflicted, you will think your reflection is somebody else."

TREATMENT

As with other misidentification disorders, Mirrored Self-Misidentification may be treated with cognitive behavioral therapy. It may eventually go away on its own, or it may require more involved treatments such as anti-psychotic medication and/or electroconvulsive therapy.

PROSOPAGNOSIA
(ALSO FACE BLINDNESS)

Because who can be expected to recognize everybody all the time . . .
or anybody, ever?

QUIZ YOURSELF

○ Do you sometimes have a difficult time recognizing old acquaintances?

○ Do you sometimes have a difficult time recognizing old friends?

○ Do you sometimes have a difficult time recognizing current friends?

○ Do you sometimes have a difficult time recognizing your spouse and children?

INNER MONOLOGUE

This is such a lovely afternoon. What a beautiful beach—the water's so blue it almost seems fake. What could possibly be wrong with a day like today? And the fact that you get to spend it with your brand-new wife, whom you love so, so much. That pushes it over the edge. This is *the* nicest day of your life. And look at that beautiful woman lying there in her pink bathing suit. She looks like a goddess in this sunlight. You get to spend the rest of your life with that woman. She actually married you. How did you pull that off?

Her legs are so soft, her thighs are so tight. Tighter than you remember. She must have been working out for the wedding. You can run your hand up her thigh. She is your wife, after all. And no one's looking.

Well now, that was a strange reaction. She's screaming. Something's wrong. People are running over. Something's definitely wrong.

Damn it! Your wife was wearing a *red* bathing suit, you idiot. You have to remember things like that. How many times are you going to let that happen?

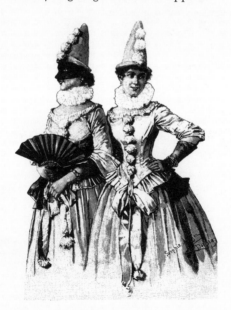

PROSOPAGNOSIA

You know that feeling you get when you run into somebody on the street, and he knows you, but you don't know him, so when he calls you by name, you have to say something like, "What's up, buddy?" As far as you know, this guy could be anybody. You study his clothes, his hair, his face for any clues to who the hell he is, imagining him against a variety of backgrounds (brick wall, forest, opium den), hoping something will spark some recognition inside your head and release you from this infuriating confusion. You know that feeling? Now imagine if it happened every time you saw *anybody*. That's Prosopagnosia.

The disorder derives its name from the Greek *prosopon*, for "face," and *agnosia*, for "I have no idea." People with Prosopagnosia literally cannot recognize people by their facial features. It in no way suggests blindness, and in fact has nothing to do with eyesight. You are simply unable to connect any information or emotion to the faces of others. It's like meeting everybody for the first time each and every time you see them.

The problem lies in the brain. When you see a thing, your eyes collect all the data about that thing (lines, curves, color, etc.). They pack it up and send it along the optical nerves to your brain, where the information is passed around and put back together in a way that makes sense. One part says, "Oh, it's a face." "A man's face," another adds. Another pipes up, "The man's face looks angry." And the area of the brain that Prosopagnosia affects says things like, "It's your friend John, whose wife you slept with." But if that part isn't working properly, you're going to miss your cue and likely get punched in the neck.

Doctors don't fully understand why this happens; Prosopagnosia often occurs following a head injury, but in many cases it occurs seemingly without cause.

TREATMENT

About half of all reported cases of Prosopagnosia resolve themselves in a few months, after the brain relearns how to transmit and process information. However, if it doesn't clear up in a few months, the chances of it ever going away are slim. You'd be wise to start paying very close attention to people's voices and the way they comb their hair.

SYNDROME OF SUBJECTIVE DOUBLES

Because even Superman has an evil twin.

QUIZ YOURSELF

- O   Do you ever think you have a doppelganger?
- O   Do you ever think you have a double?
- O   Do you ever think you have a look-alike?
- O   Do you ever think you have a person who looks just like you?

INNER MONOLOGUE

How can you just sit there when you know *he's* out there, doing God only knows what? There must be something you can do to protect your good reputation. If he happens into the wrong bar at the wrong time and meets the wrong person . . . anything could happen. He's walking around with *your face*.

Maybe you should think this through. Odds are, he's just some normal guy—like you—who happens to look *exactly like you*; he probably won't do anything terrible. Besides, these things happen. A quarter of the people in this town must have precise doubles. Seriously, how many variations on a human face can there be? Sure, you've never met two people who look *exactly* the same. Well, besides twins. And celebrity impersonators. But you're no celebrity, and this guy isn't your twin. What does he want?

Probably nothing. He's just living his life. Unless he's living *your* life. What if he's slowly supplanting you in your circle of friends? Or sidling up to the cute blonde at the record store—the one you've been laying the groundwork with for weeks . . . who *knows* what damage he could do! All your careful plotting could be undone in a few swift, ungentlemanly moves.

Or what if she likes the imposter more than she likes you?

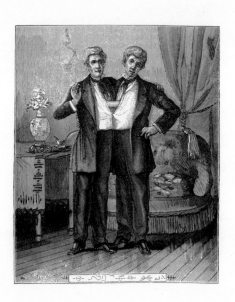

SYNDROME OF SUBJECTIVE DOUBLES

CONTINUED

DIAGNOSIS

Syndrome of Subjective Doubles is the belief that you have a doppelganger—a person who looks just like you. Once it occurs to you that this person exists, it becomes impossible to convince you otherwise. This is not an inebriated musing or the kind of thing you dreamed up on the roof of your dorm when you should have been doing philosophy homework; it's the very real belief that your double exists and is out there, waiting to ruin your good name.

You may believe that the doppelganger means you no harm. Or you may believe he has more sinister plans. The question for people with Syndrome of Subjective Doubles becomes, are you going to let him take over your life, or are you going to do something about it?

CAUSALITY

The syndrome may be caused by a psychiatric problem, such as a Delusional Disorder, or it may be caused by actual damage to the right cerebral hemisphere. This damage may be caused by anything from a stroke to Alzheimer's disease to a blunt head trauma.

> "This is not an inebriated musing or the kind of thing you dreamed up on the roof of your dorm."

TREATMENT

Treatment options vary depending on the cause. An antipsychotic drug may be helpful if the disorder is caused by a psychiatric problem. If the problem is something physically wrong inside the brain, electroconvulsive therapy may be needed.

Of Note . . .

Another, utterly charming, form of Syndrome of Subjective Doubles also exists. In this second form, rather than believing there is somebody out there who looks just like you, you believe that your brain has been removed from your head and placed into another person's.

Yep.

SYNESTHESIA

Because sometimes an apple sounds like a primary color.

QUIZ YOURSELF

- Can you see G-minor?
- Can you hear sweetness?
- Can you taste a smooth countertop?
- Can you feel cigarette smoke?
- Can you smell purple?

INNER MONOLOGUE

Oh, my God! This room is a complete disaster. What *maniac* decided mauve curtains would be palatable with a gray carpet? Whoever it was obviously had no sense of taste. So bland. So very, very bland. We'll have to redecorate in here from scratch.

Let's see, we'll start out with a deep burgundy wallpaper, something savory and rich with a slight smokiness. And then, maybe some navy-blue trim, for sweetness. And you know what would enhance that sweetness? Just a pinch of salty pink shelving. Just a pinch. And, to give it a little kick, one really spicy gold coffee table . . . right . . . there.

Ahh, this room is tasting better already.

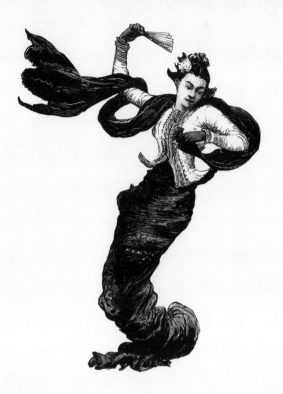

DIAGNOSIS

You know how when you look at a picture of a raging fire, your mind thinks or remembers, "hot"? Or when you push the C key of a piano, and you consider that it reminds you of the color yellow? Well, that's *not* Synesthesia. Sorry to disappoint. Here's what Synesthesia actually is: Awesome.

To be slightly more precise, Synesthesia is a mixed sensation, a blending of two or more of the five senses. If the color red is sharp and jagged, if the scent of apple pie is fluffy, if the texture of the brick wall in your in-laws' basement sounds like a pale turquoise Monday . . . that's Synesthesia. It has nothing to do with memory. It has nothing to do with any mnemonic device you invented to get yourself through piano lessons without incurring the wrath of your overbearing mother. It's an actual sensation you experience.

In fact, many "Synesthetes" aren't even aware of their condition; the syndrome is so much a part of the way their brains work, it's subconscious. If you were to fill up a piece of graph paper with little 5s with one 2 hidden in the corner, a Synesthete who considers 2s red would immediately be able to point it out.

One in 100 people experience Synesthesia regularly (hallucinogenic drugs have been known to bring upon its effects temporarily), and it is seven times more likely to occur in people with strong creative tendencies.

CAUSALITY

As desirable as it may seem, Synesthesia is technically a mental disorder, in that it's the result of something not working correctly inside your brain. Neurologists don't understand exactly why or how Synesthesia occurs, but it appears to be genetic. The most popular modern theory is that it is caused by a sort of cross-wiring inside the brain. Colors and numbers are processed in the same general region, for example, so it's not difficult to imagine a color nerve accidentally plugged into a letter receptor.

TREATMENT

Why would you possibly want to be cured of Synesthesia? It's like a superpower. Sure, there are probably some downsides to tasting music or feeling colors. But even Superman had kryptonite. So if you have Synesthesia, enjoy the positive aspects and stop complaining.

Of Note . . .

It is theorized that many of humanity's finest pieces of art were a result of Synesthesia, that its influence on painting, music, and literature is vast. Vladimir Nabokov, one of the most famous and accomplished Synesthetes, wrote in his autobiography, *Speak Memory*, that the English letter A has "the tint of weathered wood," and R is "a sooty rag bag being ripped."

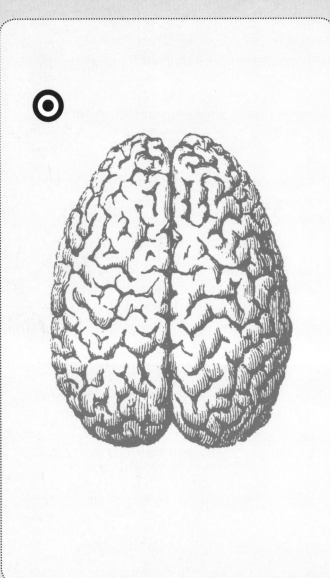

FACTITIOUS
DISORDERS

Because sometimes the mind conspires

to screw with the body.

MUNCHAUSEN SYNDROME
(ALSO FACTITIOUS DISORDER)

Because a shaved head and rigorous diet are worth the effort when the sympathy cards start rolling in.

QUIZ YOURSELF

O   Do you wrestle with feelings of depression?

O   Have you often felt lonely and in need of sympathy?

O   Do you think of the emergency room as a good place to meet girls?

O   Have you ever intentionally bled yourself to induce symptoms of anemia?

O   Do you keep minor poisons around the house just in case you really start to crave human contact?

INNER MONOLOGUE

Man, there's nothing on TV. Actually, there hasn't been anything on TV for several hours now. There must be something better to do. It sure would be nice to have somebody around to spend time with. To take care of you. To make you feel like you're not alone in the world.

You know, you do still have that vial of *Escherichia coli* bacteria lying around. You could do a little shot of that and then swing over to the hospital complaining of abdominal cramps, diarrhea, and bloody stool. The doctors and nurses would have to take care of you, it's their job!

Damn it! Where is that stupid *E. coli*?! Well, you could lop off a finger instead. You know, take the cleaver you use to carve up Costco steaks and give your pinky a good whack. Shock oughta set in before you feel too much pain, and then you're guaranteed to get medical attention. Reattachment surgery, too.

And if that doesn't work, next time you can shave your head and shoot for cancer.

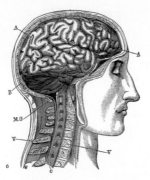

DIAGNOSIS

Victims of Munchausen Syndrome, though not physically ill to begin with, will go to incredible lengths to receive medical care—for example, starving themselves, injecting chemicals, ingesting minor poisons, or feigning seizures.

Some have gone so far as to amputate a digit. Sufferers will study symptoms so that they may expertly recreate them and fool hospital staffs into admitting them for treatment. Once there, they will happily endure whatever invasive or painful procedures follow. If cured, they will often re-induce symptoms and start over again at another hospital.

And why? Just because. For the attention. Because it's rather nice to have doctors and nurses fawning all over you, especially if you're lonely or seeking to fill an emotional hole. This is not to be confused with "malingering," in which people fake medical problems to escape responsibility or for financial gain. Still, Munchausen Syndrome can get quite expensive for the government. In fact, Washington State claims to have save about $100,000 per year by tracking repeat Munchausen patients.

CAUSALITY

Victims of this disorder often have a history of emotional or physical abuse, which bring about feelings of inadequacy and loss of identity. When faced with the myriad emotional traumas present in everyday life, they feel the overwhelming need to be tended to, to be cared for. And if nobody is around to provide the needed attention, they go out and find it on their own.

> "Even if caught in the act, they will deny, deny, deny as long as they can manage."

Treatment for Munchausen Syndrome includes antidepressants and psychotherapy, but their effectiveness is limited. Moreover, victims often have difficulty admitting to faking it—even if caught in the act, they will deny, deny, deny as long as they can manage. For this reason, very few people are cured of the disorder. For your own safety, you may be placed in long-term treatment with a mental health professional.

Of Note . . .

The disorder is named for German nobleman Karl Friedrich Hieronymus, Baron von Münchhausen (1720–1797), who was world renowned as a first-class liar. Among the very imaginative fabrications he told of his adventures—later to become the classic book *The Adventures of Baron Münchhausen*—were his riding of a bisected horse, dancing in the belly of a whale, and traveling to the moon.

FOREIGN ACCENT SYNDROME

Because it's not pretentious if you can't stop doing it.

- Are you not from a country other than the one you're from?
- Do you speak as though you were not from a country other than the one you're not from?
- If you were to speak in the accent of a country that you weren't from, would it sound like you were totally faking it?

INNER MONOLOGUE

Wot ohn Eahrth can zey be tawking ahbout? Why wohld you be taw-king wit a Frunch ak-sent? You are frum zee mid-dell ov Ken-tuck-ee? You huv ne-vear efven bean to Eu-ropp? Pay no atten-shun to zair stoo-ped blath-thur. You szound puhrfectly nor-mahl. Zey are awl jusd crdazy.

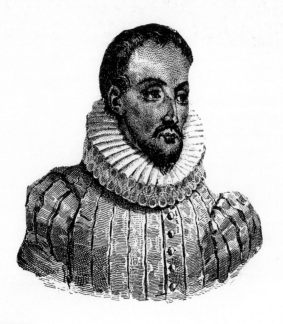

DIAGNOSIS

This really happens. Stop being so suspicious. It is 100 percent documented by medical and psychological professionals. It's extremely rare; there have been fewer than twenty documented cases in the world. But those cases were real. And several of them have occurred within the past ten years.

Oddly, in November of 1999, two separate cases were reported. One was a British woman from Kent who acquired a French accent, even though she'd only been to France once.

The other was an American woman, born in Indiana and living in Florida (but who naturally had a New York accent, just to make this all more convoluted), who suddenly found herself with a British accent, despite never having been to England.

CAUSALITY

The exact cause of this disorder is unknown. One possible explanation is that God has a sense of humor. Another explanation is that it is linked to damage in the left hemisphere of the brain, where language is processed; the two November 1999 cases both acquired Foreign Accent Syndrome following incidents of strokes. But just about any brain injury could set it off. You just never know.

It's speculated that the victim is not *actually* acquiring a foreign accent, but that the brain injury interferes with speech mechanisms, so that you end up changing your voice's pitch and lengthening or shortening your syllables in such a way that it resembles the vocal patterns of a foreign accent. And it can happen with any accent. It could be French or British or even Mortlockese. It just depends on the way your brain reacts to the tissue damage.

> ## "One possible explanation is that God has a sense of humor."

TREATMENT

Generally, Foreign Accent Syndrome goes away on its own, if you can rely on the few documented cases in which it has occurred. Speech therapy can accelerate the process. It helps to remember that some people live with foreign accents their whole lives.

Of Note...

The first documented case of Foreign Accent Syndrome occurred in a Norwegian woman in 1941. She was hit with shrapnel in the head and then suffered severe language problems. When those problems cleared up, she was left with a rather unfortunate side effect: a German accent. (In case you're not up on your World War II history, a year earlier, Norway—a neutral country—was invaded by Nazi Germany. So, the Germans weren't especially popular in the victim's neighborhood.) She was subsequently ostracized by her community.

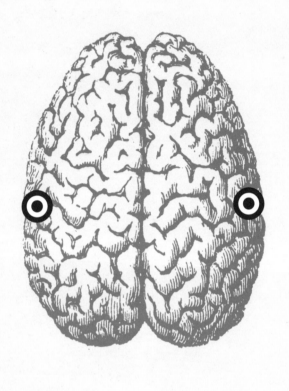

IMPULSE-CONTROL DISORDERS

Because it's possible to act without your own permission.

COMPULSIVE HOARDING
(ALSO PATHOLOGICAL HOARDING)

Because you never know when you'll absolutely need that November 4, 1985, issue of People *magazine with Cybill Shepherd on the cover.*

QUIZ YOURSELF

- O Do you enjoy collecting things?
- O Do you have a difficult time parting with old keepsakes?
- O Do you see value in objects that others don't see, be it practical or emotional?
- O Do you never, ever throw anything away?
- O Do you have a difficult time moving around inside your home?

INNER MONOLOGUE

Wait, you can't throw that away! What are you, crazy? That's a perfectly good broken wrench. Go put it on the kitchen stove with the other broken wrenches. Eventually, you're going to get around to fixing them, and then won't you be glad you saved this one?

And don't even *think* about tossing that bag of old, stained, ripped t-shirts. That would be a sin. Do you realize how many poor children there are in the world walking around with no shirts? You leave that bag right where it is. Let's not be wasteful.

Ooh . . . look at that rubber band. No way that's headed for the trash. Rubber bands are *always* useful! Go on, throw it in the bathtub with the others.

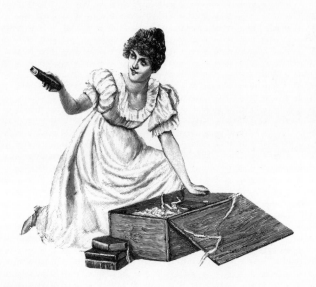

DIAGNOSIS

You know that stupid note from your ex that you can't bring yourself to throw away? It's just a scribble on the back of an envelope from the gas company asking you to pick up a jar of capers, but for some reason you've endowed it with "meaning." Maybe you even managed to drop it in the trash once, but then felt weird somehow, so you dug it out and brushed off the coffee grounds, and now it's tucked away in your dresser. That ex is several exes ago. Keeping the note doesn't really make sense, but it's a slight ridiculousness you allow yourself.

Now imagine if you placed that kind of importance on everything. A key to a door that no longer exists. A pay stub for a summer job you had back in college. An empty potato chip bag from a boxed lunch you ate on a bus one time. Imagine that you can't bring yourself to throw any of these items away. So they pile up in your home in huge teetering stacks. You run out of room on the shelves so you start new stacks on the floor and the washing machine and on top of the refrigerator. You can't sleep in your bed because it's covered in power chargers and digital clocks that no longer work but that you might need one day. You have to enter your house through the back door because the front door is blocked by boxes of old shoes. And even if there was a reason to get into the guestroom, you'd have to climb over so many issues of *Newsweek* that it wouldn't be worth the trouble.

If you can imagine that, you have a pretty good handle on what it's like to suffer from Compulsive Hoarding.

CAUSALITY

Compulsive Hoarding is commonly seen as a form of Obsessive-Compulsive Disorder; however, studies have shown differences in brain activity between the two. Compulsive Hoarding is not listed in the *Diagnostic and Statistical Manual of Mental Disorders IV* (the Bible of the psychological field), and there is little research being done on it. Regardless, you'll want to tear this page out and keep it with your stacks of potentially relevant articles, because eventually it's sure to be of some use.

TREATMENT

Here's what *not* to do: throw away all the Compulsive Hoarder's junk and then say, "Now, doesn't that feel better?" This will likely cause the sufferer to become extremely—possibly violently—angry, and may induce acute despondency.

Also, medications prescribed for people with OCD commonly don't work for Compulsive Hoarders. Cognitive behavioral therapy with a trained psychologist can help the Hoarder learn to whittle his or her collection of valuable junk, and at least reduce it to a livable level of clutter.

HYPERGRAPHIA
(ALSO GERSCHWIND SYNDROME)

Because there are all these words piling up inside your head, and you have to get some of them out.

QUIZ YOURSELF

O   Do you sometimes feel the need to express your thoughts through words?

O   Do you enjoy the act of writing?

O   If you were to find your desk had caught fire, would you be more likely to attempt to extinguish the fire or write a manifesto against fire's unfair persecution of desks?

O   Would you be willing to write a 100,000-word essay on how much you enjoy writing 100,000-word essays? Have you done this already?

O   Did you write this book?

INNER MONOLOGUE

There's still some blank space left over by the window, isn't there? Beneath the ledge, where you were writing about the eternal river of souls flowing not through people but in the space that exists *between* people. Didn't you finish that thought on the inside of the medicine cabinet? There should be just enough space on the wall for you to explain your

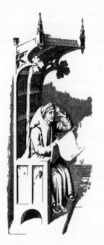

belief that entropy is not so much a destructive force as it is a reductive force, leveling all matter to a state of absolute simplicity. If you write small enough.

But your pen is pretty shot. The felt tip is so flat you'll never be able to write small enough, even if you don't cite references. Can't anyone make a decent pen anymore? Seriously. That's the three-thousandth pen you've gone through this month. You've got to find a new brand. Speaking of which, you've got to remember to restock the stash of notepads in the pantry with a fresh gross. Easier than writing on the walls.

DIAGNOSIS

Hypergraphia is the overwhelming compulsion to write. And write. And write. Once you start writing, you just can't stop. You don't want to stop. The words pour out, and your pen can barely keep up with them. Even when you run out of paper, you won't stop. There are bills on the end table. And the pizza boy left a flyer by the front door. Of course, there are rolls of nice clean paper in the bathroom too, aren't there? And if that runs out, you've always got walls, furniture, skin . . .

This desire to write and write and write doesn't always take such manic turns. You won't find every person with Hypergraphia filling his or her home with journals' worth of incredibly small scribbles. In fact, many with the disorder don't view it as a disorder at all; they think of it as a blessing. Some people make careers of their Hypergraphia, writing book after book after book. Some people with Hypergraphia write classics. However, that only occurs with people who have both Hypergraphia and talent, and the two don't necessarily coexist. For every *Crime and Punishment* there are countless volumes of *Things I Like to Write About While I Sit in My Bedroom and Write About Things I Like to Write About*.

CAUSALITY

Hypergraphia has been linked to both epilepsy and bipolar disorder. Fluctuations in brainwave activity in the temporal lobe—temporal lobe seizures, specifically—are likely to blame for the disorder's manifest symptoms. A seizure acts somewhat like an electrical power surge inside your head, causing frantic activity. With Hypergraphia, ideas, words, phrases, and bad poems about cats start to pile up. They have to go somewhere. So you write.

Most people do not seek treatment for Hypergraphia, and instead simply find outlets for their streams of consciousness. However, the conditions that may cause the disorder, such as epilepsy and bipolar disorder, may be treated with anticonvulsant drugs or, in extreme cases, brain surgery.

Of Note . . .

In her book, *The Midnight Disease*, Dr. Alice Flaherty expresses her belief that Hypergraphia is the flip-side of writer's block, which is caused by similar issues in the brain's frontal lobe, rather than the temporal lobe. She and Harvard psychologist Shelly Carson are experimenting with possible cures for writer's block, including light therapy. Studies by Austrian neuroscientists have achieved positive results by passing a magnetic wand over people's heads.

However, writers throughout history have sought more primitive and time-tested forms of self-medication. Robert Louis Stevenson's cure of choice while writing *The Strange Case of Dr. Jekyll and Mr. Hyde* was cocaine. Friedrich Nietzsche's, while writing *Beyond Good and Evil*, was syphilis.

INTERMITTENT EXPLOSIVE DISORDER
(ALSO RAGE DISORDER)

Because you have to stay calm, you have to stay calm, you have to . . .
SMASH THAT TABLE!

QUIZ YOURSELF

- O Do you find yourself easily frustrated?
- O Do your emotions sometimes get the better of you?
- O Are there holes in the plaster of your walls?

INNER MONOLOGUE

All the housework is complete, and you did a fine job. Now, it's time for you to reward yourself with a trip to the ice cream parlor to buy yourself a nice big double scoop of Rocky Road. You've earned it. Just put on your jacket. And grab those car keys.

Silly you. You dropped the car keys. Isn't that funny? One would think that if you could spend an afternoon delicately hand-wiping a collection of antique hand-painted commemorative Royal Worcester family dishes, then you could easily lift a set of crude car keys. Just grab them again and get going.

You, uh, dropped them again. Ha ha. This isn't . . .

difficult. Any three-year-old child can pick up a set of keys. It's really the most basic of motor skills. Hey, maybe you should get a three-year-old child in here to pick them up for you. That's right. Laugh it off. Now grab those keys.

Mother of [expletive deleted]!! What the [expletive deleted] is wrong with you?! How [expletive deleted] hard is it to [expletive deleted] pick up a [expletive deleted] set of [expletive deleted] keys?! Throw those [expletive deleted] keys across the room! Take that you [expletive deleted] car [expletive deleted] keys!! You can wipe down these stupid [expletive deleted] plates but you can't [expletive deleted] grab some car keys?! Oh look, all the [expletive deleted] dishes are getting smashed! You're smashing all the [expletive deleted] dishes because you don't [expletive deleted] get to have a [expletive deleted] set of [expletive deleted] dishes! Good! Take that you [expletive deleted] plates. Take that!!

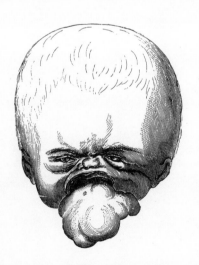

INTERMITTENT EXPLOSIVE DISORDER

CONTINUED

DIAGNOSIS

Most people have experienced moments of mild to moderate anger brought about by seemingly small examples of life's little annoyances. You break a nail, you might let fly a four-letter-word. Somebody cuts you off in traffic, you might follow him home and shave a threatening message onto his dog. Sufferers from Intermittent Explosive Disorder, however, experience this anger to a degree wildly disproportionate to the actual situation. Outbursts are punctuated by periods of verbal abuse, violence, or destruction of property, all fueled by a sense of uncontrollable rage.

After the explosion, the tension that was brewing seems to just melt away. And assuming you haven't killed anyone in your fit of anger, you'll probably feel compelled to apologize profusely and repair any structural damage. But reparations do little to reduce the chances of a repeat episode. In fact, if you happen to knock something over while cleaning up after your tantrum, the rage may quickly return.

Though the exact causes of Intermittent Explosive Disorder are unknown, imbalanced levels of the neurotransmitter serotonin are believed to play a role. The disorder is somewhat more common in men.

> "Outbursts are punctuated by periods of verbal abuse, violence, or destruction of property."

TREATMENT

Counseling through behavioral modification therapy is probably a good idea, and if the behavior persists, antidepressants and other mood-stabilizing medication may be prescribed. Being asked to sleep on the couch has also shown some positive effects.

JUMPING FRENCHMEN OF MAINE DISORDER
(ALSO LATAH)

Because you'll do what you're told, and you'll do it now.

QUIZ YOURSELF

○ Do you have a nervous or anxious temperament?
○ Do you startle easily?
○ Are you susceptible to others' commands?
○ Do you pretty much do whatever people tell you to do?

INNER MONOLOGUE

Oh no, here comes Frank. He's such a jerk. He thinks he's so funny, taking advantage of you the way he does. Well, this time, don't let him. Whatever he tells you to do, don't do it. No matter what, don't do it. Just don't listen to him. Don't pay attention to him. Just remember: don't do it. Don't do it. Don't do it. Don't do it.

Damn it! Why are you punching yourself in the face? Damn it! You're doing it! You idiot!

Well, next time. Next time you won't let him tell you what to do.

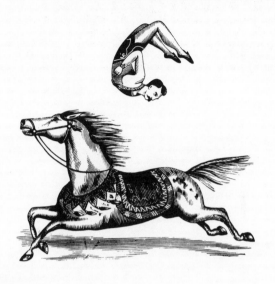

DIAGNOSIS

If somebody handed you a standard glue trap (used for catching rodents), positioned you next to your beloved mother, who carried you in her womb for nine long months, and then told you to slap the glue trap right across your mother's face, would you do it? What if he told you to in a quick, loud, and emphatic manner (a "bark," if you will)? Like hell you wouldn't. You'd do it without even thinking about it. You'd do it without even *knowing* you were doing it, and then you'd spend hours soaking your poor mother's saintly face in a bucket of soapy water, slowly, gingerly peeling the trap from her matronly wrinkles, pleading for forgiveness all the while. And do you know why? You have Jumping Frenchmen of Maine Disorder.

Jumping Frenchmen of Maine Disorder is a psychological problem in which you will do anything anybody tells you to do, as long as they deliver the command quickly, loudly, and emphatically.

CAUSALITY

Jumping Frenchmen of Maine Disorder is thought to be caused by a form of operant conditioning. That is, when you have been taught, time and again, to do what you are told without question, that way of thinking becomes hardwired into your brain. Given a particularly harsh working environment, where disobedience is strongly punished, you might find yourself susceptible. However, psychologists don't fully understand why the disorder occurs in some such conditions and not in others.

> "You will do anything anybody tells you to do, as long as they deliver the command quickly, loudly, and emphatically."

TREATMENT

So few cases of Jumping Frenchmen of Maine Disorder have been researched by professionals that little data is available on how to treat it. One could reason that cognitive behavioral therapy would prove beneficial.

Of Note . . .

The name "Jumping Frenchmen of Maine Disorder" derives from a group of French-Canadian lumberjacks in the Moosehead Lake region of Maine in whom neurologists observed an unusually quick response to verbal commands. Small populations in Southeast Asia and Yemen have since been diagnosed, and it's believed that a great number of production assistants working within the Hollywood studio system suffer from the disorder as well.

KLEPTOMANIA

Because you need that Japanese teapot even if you don't want it.

○ Do you ever feel anxious while in department stores?
○ Do you get depressed after crossing self-delineated boundaries?
○ Do you ever find yourself thinking, "That's a really ugly candy bowl . . . and I want it"?
○ Have you been arrested multiple times for shoplifting?

INNER MONOLOGUE

That has got to be the tackiest brooch ever created. Who thought it was a good idea to sculpt a pouncing leopard out of fake sapphires? And that bright orange ribbon—terrible! Even so . . . the sales lady is all the way over there, attending to that elderly woman in the Debbie Reynolds wig. She'll never see . . . Go on, grab it! Take it! It's yours!

You don't have to want it; you just have to take it. You can drop it in the parking lot once you're outside. Wouldn't it feel *good* to snatch that abominable thing? You know you want to. You can feel the tension building in your neck.

Your hand is itching. It wants that horrible leopard pin and it wants it now.

No, you can't *buy* it—totally out of the question. Just take it! That blue-and-orange piece of baublish nonsense belongs in your purse. Quick, do it before somebody's looking!

Ahh, doesn't that feel better? Okay, now go throw it out.

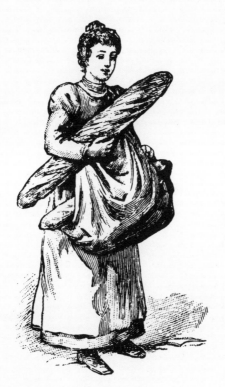

DIAGNOSIS

Kleptomania is a compulsion to steal. Victims of the disorder lack the ability to resist this compulsion, even if the object of momentary obsession is total junk—the impulse has very little to do with actual value. In fact, as often as not, the item stolen is something the victim doesn't want, and is discarded following the theft.

If you have Kleptomania, you may feel rising anxiety before stealing, and even though you know the act is wrong and will likely result in feelings of guilt, depression, and/or fear, you will find yourself unable to resist the impulse. And—just like that—some worthless piece of nothing ends up in your pocket and a security guard is following you out of the store.

CAUSALITY

Kleptomania usually develops around the age of thirty-five and occurs most frequently in women. A person may struggle with the disorder for fifteen or more years before overcoming it. While the actual causes of the disorder remain a mystery, some experts believe that it may stem from feelings of emotional shortcomings as a child. There is growing evidence, however, that it may be linked to a lack of serotonin in the brain.

> ## "And—just like that—some worthless piece of nothing ends up in your pocket."

TREATMENT

Antidepressants such as Prozac have been found useful in treating Kleptomania but should be prescribed in combination with behavior modification therapy, to help you find a tension-relieving activity to take the place of stealing.

Of Note . . .

Although Kleptomania is widely considered a valid mental disorder, it is not considered a sufficient excuse for thievery in most courtrooms. In other words, if you get caught with un-paid-for mother-of-pearl butterfly hairclips in your bag, you're on your own.

PATHOLOGICAL GAMBLING

Because any minute now your luck is going to turn, and then you can fix all the things you screwed up till now.

QUIZ YOURSELF

- O Do you like to take chances?
- O Do numbers and odds interest you?
- O Do you experience a thrill watching mechanisms of chance play themselves out?
- O Seriously, what are the chances that you're going to lose *again*?

INNER MONOLOGUE

All right, you really need to stop this way of life. Look at you, sitting in the park because you're too embarrassed to tell your wife that you lost your job because you gambled away your expense account in Atlantic City. This is too much. Enough is enough. You're stopping this now.

Here's the deal. See that little girl over there in the sundress? If she climbs up the sliding board, you're done gambling forever; if she jumps onto the spin-y thing, you go on as you've been going on. Ah, there she goes . . .

Okay, double or nothing. If that pigeon lands on the

statue, not only are you done gambling, you'll also go to church every week. If it lands on the bench, you'll proceed as normal. Damn it! Okay, this time. If that homeless guy throws up onto those two nuns, you're done gambling, you'll go to church, and you'll spend three nights a week working in a soup kitchen. There's a good one you could check out in Vegas . . .

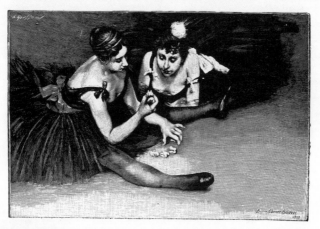

DIAGNOSIS

Everybody knows that working hard for your money is for suckers and Protestants. It's not the American way. Free money is where it's *at*. But you have to know what you're doing to get free money, and it takes a lot of work to know what you're doing. Actually, it's harder work getting your money free than working for it. But it's so much more satisfying.

And that's the allure of gambling. The patter of tumbling dice. The flitter of shuffling cards. The squawking of tussling roosters. These sounds cut right to the heart and stir up feelings that can't be replicated by any other activity. It's like a drug. And it's not just the money—it's the chance, the risk. Luck itself can be as strong and satisfying a drug as heroin. And just as addictive.

For approximately ten million Americans today, gambling is more than a means of entertainment or a thing to do besides waiting by the phone for their grandchildren to call. It's the centerpiece of their lives. They sink entire paychecks into Blackjack and Poker and that game the taxi drivers are always playing. They can't help themselves. Betting rent and winning it back 3–1 feels great. Amazing and euphoric. But not as great as the next bet. And the one after that. For these people, it's about the playing more than the winning, which is good, because if you play long enough, you're going to lose. The odds are against you. (Casinos and bookies are smart that way.) And when you lose your rent money, what do you do? You try to win it back. So you bet next month's rent. And what do you do when you lose that? And if you win it back what do you do? It doesn't matter; you're going to keep betting anyway. That's Pathological Gambling.

Pathological Gamblers are incapable of *not* gambling. It's not simply a matter of poor judgment or a lack of respect for money; it's a genuine psychological addiction. And it can be just as damaging to the victims' lives and their family's lives as a drug addiction.

> ## "And when you lose your rent money, what do you do? You try to win it back."

TREATMENT

Cognitive behavioral therapy may be helpful in getting Pathological Gamblers to seek pleasure in more fruitful ventures. Like knitting. Knitting can be just as exciting as gambling, particularly when you start getting into the philosophical differences between Beaded Knitting and Bead Knitting. They sound pretty much the same, but, oh man—they're not.

PICA

Because if you can get it in your mouth, you can eat it.

- O   Do you enjoy eating dirt?
- O   How about clay?
- O   How about hair?
- O   Glue? Chalk? Wax? Chewing gum? Foam rubber?
      Toothpicks? Matchsticks? Coat buttons? Pen caps?
      Wrapping paper? Glass shards?
- O   Human feces?

INNER MONOLOGUE

What's it to them if you feel like eating rubber bands? You're a grown-up. You make your own decisions. You can eat all the rubber bands you want. In fact, if you want to eat a bag of rubber bands for breakfast, then another two for lunch and three more for dinner, it's your Constitutional right to do so! Your forefathers bled to death in icy ditches with musket pellets in their chest so that you could eat rubber bands for every single meal if you so choose.

So what if they say rubber bands have no nutritional value? It's all relative, isn't it? Like, who really knows? Doctors are always changing their minds about food and nutrition and stuff. Maybe in thirty years, yuppies will be swallowing huge bowls full of rubber bands. There could be entire restaurants dedicated to serving rubber bands of different lengths and consistencies. Different grades of rubber. Different widths! Mmmm, widths. You're getting hungry.

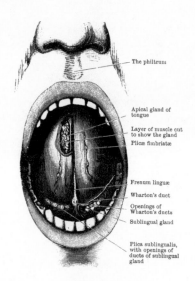

The philtrum

Apical gland of tongue

Layer of muscle cut to show the gland

Plicæ fimbriatæ

Frenum linguæ

Wharton's duct

Openings of Wharton's ducts

Sublingual gland

Plica sublingualis, with openings of ducts of sublingual gland

DIAGNOSIS

Strictly speaking, a compulsion to eat non-nutritive materials is not considered "normal" behavior by the psychiatric community. And while many forms of Pica are completely benign, others pose minor, serious, or idiotic health risks. Eating dirt by the handful, for example, probably won't kill you, but it may contain bacteria that doesn't sit well with your digestive tract—a minor health risk. Eating feces poses considerably more danger, placing it in the "serious risk" category. Eating rusty razor blades dipped in poison, it then follows, is an idiotic health risk.

Pica sufferers would be wise to remember one basic fact of human consumption: What goes in must come out. And it's a *long* way from here to there. Approximately thirty feet of pipeline connect the mouth to the anus, and an unwisely swallowed bolt can do a lot of damage to the plumbing. Various objects may produce such unwanted effects as gastric pain, constipation, bowel perforation, kidney damage, and/or mental retardation. (A word to the wise: Paint chips are not a snack food.)

CAUSALITY

In certain cases, Pica may be associated with nutritional deficiencies. It has been found that many people who eat clay, for example, are iron deficient, though doctors are unsure which factor is cause and which is effect.

Some theorize that Pica may be caused by a lack of dopamine, a chemical that controls the flow of impulses inside the brain. No evidence for this currently exists, but if the evidence was found and subsequently written down on a piece of paper, it may have been eaten.

> ## "A word to the wise: Paint chips are not a snack food."

TREATMENT

Aside from being treated for the various side effects of eating non-nutritive materials, you may want to seek counseling to help you get over the disorder. (Assuming you *want* to stop eating non-nutritive materials.) Behavior modification therapy is a commonly prescribed approach.

Of Note . . .

Eating at fast food restaurants does not constitute Pica, though it technically depends on what you eat at them.

PYROMANIA

Because fire is hot.

○ Do you own more than twelve lighters?

○ Do you scour the morning paper for local fire department reports while drinking your coffee?

○ Do you ever pull your car over and spend hours rapturously watching a house burn down?

○ When you start forest fires, and witness the initial glowing embers rise up in dancing tongues of energy, does it temporarily fill a void in your sad and lonely existence?

INNER MONOLOGUE

Will you just look at that? Trees in every direction, as far as the eye can see. Absolutely breathtaking. Wow, this is really stirring something up inside you. It's hard not to be inspired in the middle of all this beauty. You need to create something.

You need to start a fire!

Not a big fire. Just a humble little thing. A light burning. Over by that really tall tree. That would complete this scene.

Nothing wrong with that, right? Fire is a naturally occurring phenomenon. A fire could start even if you weren't here. And what a bummer it would be if nobody were here to see that kind of nature interacting with nature. Hey, and people are a naturally occurring phenomenon as well. So, if you started a fire, that would just be nature setting nature upon nature. In fact, if you *didn't* start a fire, it would be an insult to natural order.

That would just be nature standing around nature not starting a fire, which is not any fun at all.

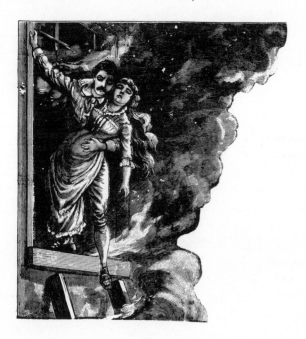

DIAGNOSIS

What is fire, exactly? We can see it and feel it, but it's not technically matter. Scientists of the past, who were very stupid, believed it was one of the four elements from which the universe was formed. Many religions, such as Judaism, Catholicism, and Hinduism, regularly use fire to burn things and curry favor from their Gods. (Whether this works or not remains in question.) One thing we definitely do know about fire is that it's awesome. There's hardly a person on Earth who doesn't use fire in some fashion every day of his or her life. We need it. And yet it can destroy your home and melt all your vintage punk-rock LPs in a matter of minutes. And because of that, it's fascinating.

If you suffer from Pyromania, this fascination is usually coupled with deep loneliness or sadness. Flame inherently appeals to you as an antidote to such cold, dark feelings. Setting a fire and watching it burn—knowing you gave birth to such a beautiful and hypnotic creature—produces a sense of euphoria. Pyromaniacs begin to crave this high and may find it difficult to recreate by any means other than starting fires.

Doctors don't know exactly what causes Pyromania. Certainly, depression and loneliness play a role, but if that were all, there would be a lot more burning houses right now. Some psychologists believe that Pyromania may be a malformed attempt at communication in people with poor social skills.

TREATMENT

The usual course of treatment for Pyromania is behavior modification therapy, though results here are mixed. It's essential that the Pyromaniac learn to channel his or her feelings of sadness and loneliness into something more constructive than fire, such as anything else.

Of Note . . .

Many Pyromaniacs become excited by anything associated with fire, including firefighters at work. If you happen to frequent house burnings just to watch the firefighters do their thing, you may notice the same people standing beside you in the crowd time and again. There's a good chance many of those familiar faces—yours included—are Pyromaniacs to some degree.

IMPULSE–CONTROL DISORDERS

TRICHOTILLOMANIA

Because ripping out your own hair is better than being frantically consumed with the urge to rip out your own hair.

QUIZ YOURSELF

- ○ Do you sometimes feel overwhelmed by minutia?
- ○ Do you crave a means to release mounting stress?
- ○ Do you have bald patches on your scalp, eyebrows, or pubic area?
- ○ Have you ever torn a clump of hair from your body and shoved the dismembered strands into your mouth?

INNER MONOLOGUE

That report needs to be on the boss's desk by Monday morning, which shouldn't be a problem, right? You've done all the research and there are only a few numbers left to be crunched. Converting them into a spreadsheet should be a cakewalk. Still, though, something could go wrong . . .

Come to think of it, maybe there's something you're forgetting, some vital datum that's going ignored. And what if there's a hard-drive crash? Have you backed up your information? Have you backed up your backup? What if there's a fire? All that hard work will be for nothing. You'll be a failure; you'll let everyone down. The department will fall behind its quarterly goals. There'll be layoffs. Everyone will hate you.

Okay. There's only one thing to do. Reach up, wrap your fingers around a tuft of hair, and rip it out. Forget that you swore you wouldn't do it anymore. Forget the spreading patch of baldness. This is an emergency! People will be jumping from windows, and it'll all be your fault! Do it! Rip out that hair! It has to come out! Now!!

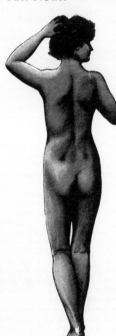

Ahh . . . That's better, isn't it? Don't you feel calmer now? One quick jerk, and all the pressure melts away. Go on, brush that freshly torn lock across your cheek. Part your lips and let the hair tickle the sides of your tongue. It's all going to be okay. None of that bad stuff will happen. Everything is fine.

Unless . . . Did you leave the oven on at home?

TRICHOTILLOMANIA

CONTINUED

DIAGNOSIS

Trichotillomania is a form of Obsessive-Compulsive Disorder in which the common stresses of daily life drive sufferers to literally tear their hair out. Once the hair has been yanked, victims experience a short period of relief from stress, as if a pressure valve has been opened (though it's likely to build up again shortly).

Sufferers of the disorder may pull the hair one follicle at a time, or rip out entire clumps. The hair may come from the scalp, eyebrows, eyelashes, or even the pubic region. Additionally, they may find pleasure in fondling the hair and, in rare cases, even sucking on it.

Because hair is usually pulled out by the root, bald patches will soon begin to form, often leading to embarrassment, shame, and more stress—stress that can be quelled (momentarily) by pulling out more hair.

CAUSALITY

Though depression or trauma may trigger episodes of Trichotillomania, they are generally not believed to be the cause of the problem. Many psychological experts are beginning to believe the disorder is brought about by a disruption in the chemical messengers in the nerve cells of the brain.

TREATMENT

Although drugs such as Anafranil, Prozac, and lithium are sometimes prescribed to control compulsive hair pulling-out, these yield limited results. A behavioral treatment known as Habit Reversal Training has proven more effective. Patients may slowly overcome Trichotillomania by understanding when and why they are compelled to pull out their hair, and then by replacing it with another activity.

Of Note . . .

Some with Trichotillomania will also indulge in Trichophagia, a form of Pica (page 116) in which the hair that was recently pulled out is swallowed. In some cases, this leads to a medical condition called Rapunzel Syndrome. Since the human body is not equipped to digest hair, a trichobezoar (wad of hair) may accumulate in the digestive tract, causing intestinal blockage and requiring surgical removal. Imagine a hairball, like those pulled from your shower drain—pulled from your colon.

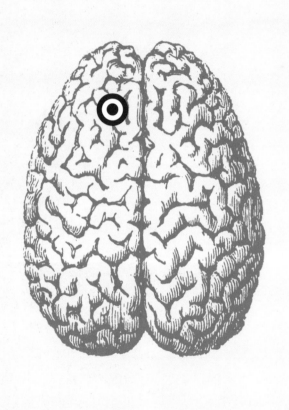

PERSONALITY
DISORDERS

Because they don't call it a superego for nothing.

EROTOMANIA
(ALSO DE CLERAMBAULT'S SYNDROME, OLD MAID'S PSYCHOSIS)

Because you can make him love you if you just try hard enough.
And if you can get near him.

QUIZ YOURSELF

○ When in love, do you find yourself going overboard to impress the object of your desire?
○ Do you ever fall for people who are "out of your league"?
○ Do you have obsessive qualities?
○ Do you know the best place to buy high-power binoculars and other surveillance equipment?
○ Have you ever sent a human organ through the U.S. Postal Service?

INNER MONOLOGUE

What's this? Did you leave the saltshaker here on the counter? Didn't you actually leave it over here, just slightly to the left of where it is now? Yes, thought so! He must have been here. The air even *smells* like he was here. God, it's almost embarrassing how much he's into you. Jetting away from his mansion in London just to climb through your window and move the saltshaker to let you know how much he loves you, and how he's going to leave his supermodel fiancée as soon as the time is right to come sweep you off your feet.

Still, it would be nice if he would call. Or at least leave a note. This whole saltshaker business is a little cold, especially since he's so madly in love with you. Even last week, when he sprinkled your television set with dust to tell you he dreams about caressing your thighs, that was better. Sure, he can't risk the news getting out to the tabloids that he's finally found his one and only. That would put undue pressure on your relationship before it had a chance to blossom into the passionate affair it will undoubtedly someday become.

This waiting gets a little tiresome, though. Oh well. It should be happening any day now.

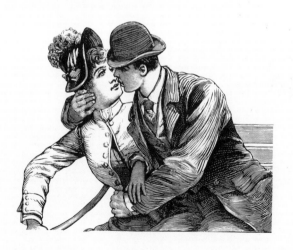

DIAGNOSIS

Erotomania is the delusional belief that someone, usually of a higher status or social order, is in love with you. The person doesn't actually have to know you, or have met you, or even exist in the real world. None of that matters, because love conquers all logic.

If you suffer from Erotomania, chances are you're not exactly loving it. It is *extremely* unlikely that the object of your obsession will pull his limo in front of your house and emerge with a bouquet of roses and the promise of undying love. As time passes, you may become embittered and paranoid. Moved to act, you may attend a concert or movie premiere headlined by your loved one and endeavor to make eye contact. You may camp out in the parking lot of his hotel, get shooed away by police, and then return to camp out again. Driven to extremes, you may then mail a human finger to his publicist to symbolize how his singing voice has touched you. It may or may not be your finger.

CAUSALITY

The majority of people with Erotomania are middle-aged women who are somewhat isolated in their lives, but it can affect men as well—middle-aged men who are somewhat isolated in their lives. Socially well-adjusted individuals will generally not have the time or the desire to stalk celebrities.

The disorder is often brought upon by larger psychiatric problems such as Paranoid Schizophrenia, which impairs your ability to perceive reality properly, or Narcissistic Personality Disorder (page 138).

TREATMENT

The problem with treating a person who does not accurately perceive reality is that in their view of reality, they don't need help. In many cases, court-mandated treatment becomes necessary. Anti-psychotic drugs and antidepressants may be prescribed, along with psychiatric therapy.

Of Note . . .

One of the most famous victims of Erotomania was John Hinkley, Jr. In 1981, Hinkley shot President Reagan in an assassination attempt intended to impress actress Jodie Foster, who totally had a thing for Hinkley, despite the fact that she'd never met, seen, or heard of him.

Hinkley's plan, for the record, didn't work.

PERSONALITY DISORDERS

HISTRIONIC PERSONALITY DISORDER

Because you're never too old to act like a teenager at theater camp.

QUIZ YOURSELF

○ Are you flirtatious?
○ Do you like getting compliments on your looks?
○ Do you enjoy being the center of attention?
○ Can you not stand not being the center of attention?
○ Is this whole book about you?

INNER MONOLOGUE

This is outrageous. How dare he? Really! Does he think that you're going to take a slight like this lying down? This will not stand. It cannot stand. You'll get even. You have to. You've been pushed to the edge. What kind of woman does he think you are? Doesn't he realize that you are a strong, intelligent, independent, incredible woman? Can't he see that? He must be able to. Everybody knows.

So, why is he talking to that pudgy girl with the braces and the bad hair instead of you? You're so much prettier than her.

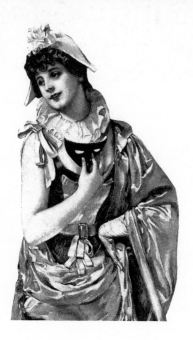

DIAGNOSIS

People with Histrionic Personality Disorder are everybody's favorite people. For about three minutes. If you
go around batting your eyelashes and thrusting your
chest at every person you meet, you are going to draw
attention, and that's exactly what you want. Because if
people aren't paying attention to you, then they might
be paying attention to somebody else. And you can't
have that.

So you'll laugh extra loudly at all their jokes to
show how engaged you are, and you'll make a big deal

of feigning empathy and listening to whatever it is they're talking about just to pull them in and capture their undivided interest.

Failing that, you may well throw a temper tantrum. Because to the Histrionic sufferer, lack of attention from others triggers extreme anxiety and agitation, and you'll take any means necessary to reduce such discomfort.

CAUSALITY

It's theorized that Histrionic Personality Disorder may develop due to a lack of parental attention as a child. Sufferers grow up seeking that attention from everybody else, at all costs. Another theory is that no theory really explains it; it's just something that develops, like expert driving skills or immaculate intuition about strangers at parties.

"Sufferers grow up seeking that attention from everybody else, at all costs."

Good luck trying to get somebody with Histrionic Personality Disorder into a psychologist's office. Why should they seek treatment? They're all so great. Once they're in there, though, they'll soon find out how great it is. Imagine, a person whose job it is to pay attention to them exclusively for an entire session. That's money well spent.

Of Note . . .

The notion of Histrionic Personality Disorder is derived from a medical problem considered by ancient Greeks called "Hysteria" or "Wandering Womb." They theorized that extreme emotions in women were caused by a displaced uterus. This theory was later dismissed in favor of a new theory that mental problems in women were caused by demonic possession and witchcraft. Both of these ideas are patently ridiculous; more likely, mental problems are caused by high-carb diets.

NARCISSISTIC PERSONALITY DISORDER

*Because you are the fulcrum around which the rest of the world spins,
and anyone who doesn't understand this is an idiot.*

QUIZ YOURSELF

- O Do you often feel underappreciated?
- O Do you have a high opinion of yourself?
- O Do you put your needs and feelings above
  those of others?
- O Do other people even have needs and feelings?
- O Are you the most important being in the universe?

INNER MONOLOGUE

What is wrong with these people? How can they all just sit there and listen to that guy prattle on? Can't they see that you're wearing a brand new shirt? And such a nice shirt, in such a nice, subtle shade of blue—"Horizon Blue," the salesman called it—that really brings out your eyes and bespeaks a refined taste in garmenture. Why is nobody complimenting you on your excellent taste?

Wait! That lady over there with the veil—she may have looked over. Did she? The least she could do is give a thumbs-up for the shirt. No, there she goes, turning back to that boring minister and his incessant, depressing eulogies. Okay, we get it. The lady's dead. That's sad, but no amount of wailing is going to bring her back. Why doesn't everyone just get over it and focus on something good in life? Like this terrific shirt?

These morons wouldn't know a nice shirt if it wrapped its sleeves around their necks and squeezed the life out of their worthless bodies. How can you expect imbeciles like them to comprehend your acute sense of style? *Why won't they notice?!*

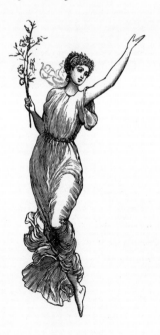

NARCISSISTIC
PERSONALITY
DISORDER CONTINUED

While everyone exhibits a certain amount of narcissism, those with full-blown Narcissistic Personality Disorder exhibit extreme selfishness and egomania. People with the disorder will harbor convictions that they are the smartest, the most attractive, the most talented, the best driver, the best orderer of seafood at Red Lobster . . . the best at whatever pursuit they choose. They will use others for personal gain and adopt an ever-changing morality to suit their needs. Often, they will lie, inventing facts or expert opinions to back up whatever they say or want.

If you think you may have Narcissistic Personality Disorder, you probably don't. However, if you think that you don't have it, there is at least a moderate chance that you do, as you will tend to disavow the possibility that you may be flawed, despite the very real probability that the disorder is rooted in a repressed feeling of inferiority. When faced with the idea that people may not want to feel subservient to your greater understanding of everything, you may at some level suffer feelings of emptiness and humiliation, but since you can't allow yourself to admit such imperfections, you'll repress them, and they will feed your narcissism. If the ego is bruised badly enough, you may strike back with rage.

CAUSALITY

Some experts theorize that the narcissistic/repressed-inferiority tendencies spring from unmet emotional needs during infancy. Others posit they arise due to some sort of abuse or trauma sustained during the first seven years of childhood.

TREATMENT

Because the roots of Narcissistic Personality Disorder likely extend back to infancy, there is little that can be done to "cure" it. The near impossibility of getting a narcissist to admit personal fault renders the question of treatment somewhat moot.

Of Note...

The term "narcissistic" comes from the Greek tale of Narcissus, whose self-love was so great that he ultimately drowned trying to get a closer look at his reflection in a pond. Had he survived, Narcissus would have pointed out that the pond's appearance was drastically improved by the presence of his beautiful corpse.

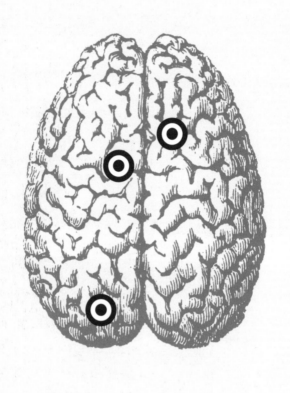

PSYCHOTIC
DISORDERS

Because sometimes the mind just snaps.

JERUSALEM SYNDROME

Because when Jesus said he'd return, he didn't say he wouldn't come back as you.

INNER MONOLOGUE

What a beautiful place this is! Boy, they don't call it the City of Gold for nothing. It's as if it's shimmering with some otherworldly light! And there are so many things to do here—how will you fit them all in? Let's see . . . you'll definitely have to go to the Israel Museum and check out the Dead Sea Scrolls. And the Phasael at the Tower of David—can't miss that. And then there are all the restaurants! Darna is supposed to be good if you like Moroccan. Or maybe just Norman's for a cheeseburger.

Then, after lunch, it's time to head back to the hotel to take your ninth shower of the day, shave all the hair from your body and drape yourself in bed sheets so that you can march down the Via Dolorosa, screaming Bible hymns into the open air, and take your place before the Church of the Holy Sepulchre, where you will deliver your heartfelt incoherent sermon to confused fellow tourists.

Ooh, don't forget to pick up a Stations of the Cross t-shirt on your way back.

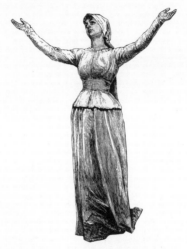

DIAGNOSIS

Jerusalem Syndrome is a phenomenon in which seemingly normal people behave in a rather overtly non-normal fashion while visiting the city of Jerusalem in Israel. The syndrome usually involves anxiety, agitation, a compulsive need to purify yourself, dressing in quasi-Biblical garb (bed sheets, animal skins, etc.), and shrill proselytizing. And since most people have only a cursory understanding of the mechanics of theological philosophy, the rants of syndrome victims often lack coherence.

Some with the syndrome actually believe themselves to be Biblical figures, such as John the Baptist, the Virgin Mary, or Jesus Christ himself. Most without the syndrome believe those people to be loud and annoying. (The sufferers of the syndrome, not the Biblical figures.) (Usually.)

CAUSALITY

Many victims of Jerusalem Syndrome have a history of psychiatric problems (in which case, technically, it's just Psychosis and could just as easily be considered St. Louis Syndrome or Tallahassee Syndrome, depending on location). But true sufferers have no history of mental disorder. You arrive at the airport, check into your hotel, and before you know it you're wearing a loincloth, flailing your arms in front of some old church.

What is generally a constant is that victims tend to come from a strong religious background, usually Protestant Christian, or, less often, Jewish. In rare cases, it affects

Catholics. Since there have also been cases in other cities with strong religious significance (Mecca, Rome, Nashville), it is thought to occur because the victim is overwhelmed with spiritual fervor in the face of what he or she believes to be genuinely holy.

TREATMENT

The syndrome should resolve itself whenever you leave the city. Many tour guides in Jerusalem have learned to recognize the warning signs, such as when a tourist expresses a desire to break away from the group and head off alone. If yours is spotted early, you may be asked to visit a hospital for psychiatric evaluation, so that any injuries or linen theft may be averted.

Of Note . . .

In 1969, an Australian tourist named Michael Rohan, apparently suffering from Jerusalem Syndrome, attempted to burn down the al-Aqsa Mosque in East Jerusalem, an act that sparked citywide riots. Rohan claimed to be acting as "the Lord's emissary" to hasten the second coming of Jesus Christ. It is still not clear whether the plan worked, since Jesus never said what time he was coming in the first place.

SHARED PSYCHOTIC DISORDER (ALSO INDUCED DELUSIONAL DISORDER, FOLIE À DEUX)

Because sometimes believing is seeing.

QUIZ YOURSELF

○ Do you share certain beliefs with other people?

○ Are some of your beliefs somewhat, shall we say, uncommon?

○ Are you close to someone who has been diagnosed with a Psychotic Disorder?

INNER MONOLOGUE

How could you have ever doubted your mother to begin with? When she first told you about the disco gnomes living in the basement, you were so quick to dismiss her warnings as crazed ramblings. You told her she'd been cooped up in this house for too long. You explained to her that gnomes are mythical creatures common to German folklore, and not real beings. You explained that gnomes are Earth spirits, so even if they did exist, they'd be living out in the wilderness, not in the basement of somebody's home. And why in the world would they be disco dancing?

But goddamnit if that's not a funky little erdgeist shaking his moneymaker right there next to the water heater. Where did he find a studded leisure suit in his size?

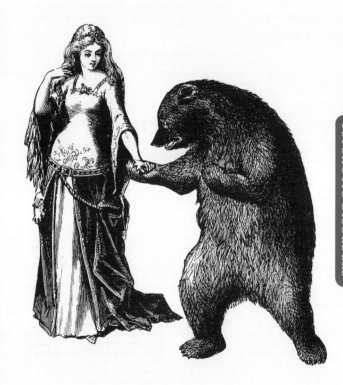

SHARED PSYCHOTIC DISORDER

CONTINUED

DIAGNOSIS

In the most common form of Shared Psychotic Disorder, in which two people share the same hallucinations and/or delusional (often paranoid) beliefs, there is usually one primary case and one secondary case. The primary case is quite often suffering from some form of Psychotic Disorder, such as Schizophrenia. The secondary case, otherwise mentally healthy, will become "infected" by the other person's psychosis.

CAUSALITY

It's not known exactly what causes a mentally well person to adopt another's psychotic beliefs, but it has been found to occur primarily between people who are tightly emotionally bound and living in relative social isolation.

"The otherwise mentally healthy will become 'infected' by the other person's psychosis."

Usually, the secondary case of a Shared Psychotic Disorder episode will return to his or her senses sometime after being separated from the primary case. If not, however, counseling through psychotherapy and possibly a short-term medication with anti-psychotics or sedatives should prove effective.

The primary case—who technically doesn't have a Shared Psychotic Disorder, but rather a Psychotic Disorder—would most likely be treated with long-term psychotherapy and anti-psychotic medication.

Of Note . . .

In rare instances, a vast number of people may suffer from the same case of Shared Psychotic Disorder. One of the more common large-scale Shared Psychotic Disorders is Penis Panic or Koro (page 170), but this *Folie à Plusieurs* ("Madness of Many") may also possibly account for the late-seventeenth-century Salem Witch Trials.

It is also believed by many that in early-November of 2004, approximately one-half of the United States suffered from a *Folie à Plusieurs*, although whether the exact percentage of the affected population was 50.7% or 49.3% depends on whom you ask.

WINDIGO PSYCHOSIS

Because there's no better cure for a boring winter evening than transforming yourself into a demonic ice spirit and hitting the town for a cannibalistic feeding frenzy.

QUIZ YOURSELF

- ○ Do you dislike the prospect of going hungry?
- ○ Do you notice changes in your own behavior when cut off from society for long periods of time?
- ○ Do you worry that you are possessed by an evil spirit?
- ○ Have you ever killed and eaten a human being?

INNER MONOLOGUE

So hungry. So hungry. You need food. This is too much. You won't be able to last much longer like this. At least if you were in town you would have people around to distract you. Of course, if you were in town, you'd probably also have food. And if you had food you wouldn't be hungry and you wouldn't need food, so you wouldn't need to be in town.

Well, you're not totally alone out here. You have your wife here with you. She can keep you occupied. You love your wife. Your beautiful wife. Your beautiful succulent wife. Your beautiful succulent delicious wife. Your succulent delicious steak. You love your steak so much. Rare. No, medium rare. Steak. Love your steak.

Hang on a second. Were you just imagining your wife as a steak? You were. You know better than that. You should never imagine your steak as a steak. Steak. Eat steak.

Listen to yourself. You're turning into a goddamn Windigo. That's all you need while you're starving out here in the wilderness, to turn into a cannibalistic demon. Just your luck. Well, if you're turning into a demon flesh-eater, there's nothing you can do about it. You might as well get crackin' on that steak. It's not going to devour itself.

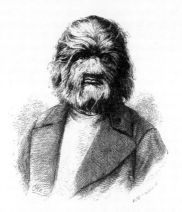

DIAGNOSIS

The Windigo, according to Anishinaabe Native American folklore, is a demon spirit with a cadaverous form and a penchant for eating people. As you can imagine, should the

WINDIGO PSYCHOSIS

CONTINUED

Windigo enter your body, it's bad news for you. As you can further imagine, it's worse news for anybody who happens to be near you. Luckily, there is no such thing as a Windigo, so the chances of actual possession are slim.

Good luck convincing Windigo Psychotics of this, though. The disorder is marked by a paranoid belief that you are possessed by or are turning into a Windigo, or indeed already are one. It begins with depression, nausea, and loss of appetite for normal (non-human-flesh-based) food. Eventually, you'll begin to see your friends and family as edible, a shift in perception followed by full psychosis and finally utter chaos, with you running around trying to kill and eat people and them running away from you screaming and crying and the police showing up with their guns out looking very concerned that this might end badly.

CAUSALITY

If you weren't raised in a culture familiar with the Windigo myth—namely the Chippewa, Cree, and Ojibwa tribes of Northern America and Canada—this probably isn't going to happen to you. But that doesn't mean you're safe from being eaten by somebody who was. As the myth goes, you can become possessed by a Windigo by happening across one in the forest at night or by simply dreaming about one.

Essentially, it's quite easy to become possessed by a Windigo. Or, to think you've been.

Windigo Psychosis occurs most frequently in famine and isolation conditions. For whatever reason, when people are cut off from society, and meanwhile grow hungry and increasingly desperate, they tend to get a little . . . cannibalistic. Experts are looking into the phenomenon.

TREATMENT

If you can calm down a Windigo Psychotic long enough to get something down his or her throat (without being eaten), bear fat has long been the medicine of choice among cultures affected. (Bear fat is rich in essential vitamins.) Minimally, getting any food into the victim is likely to help.

Of Note . . .

It is believed that when a person "becomes" a Windigo, his or her heart turns to ice. There are unsubstantiated reports of "cured" Windigo Psychotics vomiting up chunks of ice before returning to their normal, friendly, non-cannibalistic state. The fact that this is the least disturbing aspect of the disorder really says something.

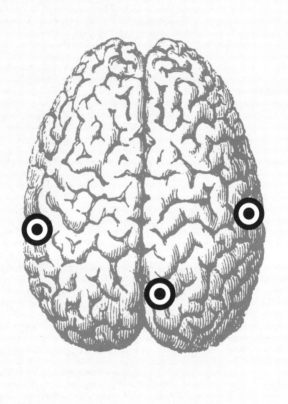

SEXUAL DISORDERS

Because sex is the doorway

to a thousand neuroses.

FROTTEURISM (ALSO FROTTAGE)

Because a day without grinding your crotch against a random stranger on the subway is like a day without sunshine.

QUIZ YOURSELF

○ Do you yearn for physical human contact?

○ Does the brush of another person's body against your own send waves of pleasure throughout your being?

○ Is it so wrong to believe that physical contact is elementally human?

○ Do you sometimes just want to rub your balls against whoever's closest to you?

INNER MONOLOGUE

Look at that girl over by the bar in the red skirt with the black tank top. Wow. She really is something. The kind of girl you can tell your grandkids about someday. All right, play it cool. Confidence is key. Just finish that beer and nonchalantly go up to the bar near her. Be smooth; remember, you're Cary Grant, you're Brad Pitt. Then, when she's not looking, rub your balls up against her.

Come on, you know you want to. What do you mean, it's wrong? Why is it wrong? She'll barely feel anything, and you'll get to go home knowing you grazed your testicles across her thigh. Everybody wins. Well, except her. But she doesn't lose that much.

It's not pathetic. How many great men were ball-rubbers? You don't know. Can you honestly say, without a doubt, that Winston Churchill never rubbed his balls against anyone in a crowded bar?

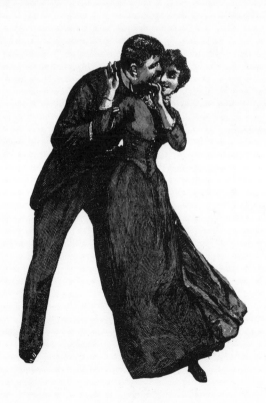

FROTTEURISM

CONTINUED

DIAGNOSIS

Just about everybody can agree that rubbing your groinal region against another person is one of the greatest pleasures with which God has seen fit, in His wisdom, to bless us. However, there are certain socially accepted prerequisites to this behavior, sometimes called dating. If you just go ahead and do it on your own without permission, it's called Frotteurism.

People with Frotteurism derive sexual pleasure from rubbing their genitals against other people without consent. Often, they will attempt this in crowded areas, such as bars, subways, or sporting events. Although it may seem to be a harmless—if, perhaps, a tad pathetic and creepy—way to get a jolt of sexual excitement, it is a recognized Paraphilia, or sexually-related mental disorder. The jury is *not* out on this one. Non-consensual sexual contact is always bad news.

CAUSALITY

The general consensus concerning the cause of Frotteurism is essentially that something is simply "off." It may stem from an experience in which the sufferer accidentally brushed his genitals against an attractive female in a crowded elevator and enjoyed it, assumed the act harmless, and kept on doing it.

Frotteurism—like all Paraphilias—is primarily a male disorder.

TREATMENT

More often than not, people won't seek treatment for Frotteurism. But if forced into treatment—by, say, a court order—psychotherapy and/or behavior modification therapy may be prescribed to uncover the root cause and replace the behavior pattern with a more socially appropriate one. Failing that, medroxyprogesterone (a female hormone) may be prescribed to decrease the sexual impulse.

Of Note . . .

Although rarely brought to trial, Frotteurism is considered a criminal offense in . . . well, just about everywhere.

INFANTILISM
(ALSO ADULT BABY SYNDROME)

Because having to act like an adult sucks anyway.

QUIZ YOURSELF

○ Do you enjoy feeling or pretending to be younger than your actual age?
○ Do you like to be coddled and cared for?
○ Do you find getting spanked during sex pleasurable?
○ Do you often dress in children's clothing?
○ Including diapers?

INNER MONOLOGUE

He needs the report by when? Three o' clock? But you've got meetings until 2:00, and you were supposed to have a phone session with your ex-wife and her man-hating "empowerment therapist" at 2:30. Yeah, that's going to be fun. You'll never get the report to your boss on time at this rate, and you know how violent he gets over missed deadlines. You've still got the bruises to show for it.

Damn it! You just spilled coffee all over your notes, and now you can't make out whether it says "Larry Rickson" or "Harry Dickson." What was that stupid guy's name? Damn it all.

You know, when this day is over, you owe yourself. Big time. Kick back with a bottle. Warm, just the way you like it. Slip into a soft, comfortable diaper, pull on your Winnie the Pooh bib and a pair of cotton booties. Maybe play a little "Farmer in the Dell" on the ol' Fisher-Price 825, and fall peacefully to sleep with your best pal Tickle Me Elmo. Elmo understands. He's the only one in this cesspool of a city who really cares about you. Elmo loves you.

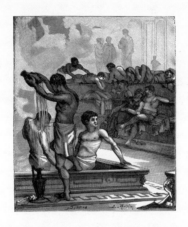

DIAGNOSIS

There are two personality types that enjoy dressing up as and acting like babies. The first, Diaper Lovers, love diapers—and, more specifically, love having sex in diapers. The second, Adult Babies, fantasize about *being* an infant.

Adult Babies are primarily heterosexual men. They do not think they're babies; they just like to pretend they are. Accordingly, if you are an Adult Baby, you may enjoy wearing not only diapers but also baby's clothing in general, as well as behaving in a babylike manner. This may include crying, crawling, rattling, chewing on action figure limbs, doing that thing where you lie on your back and wave your arms and legs in the air, eating pureed carrots, and, yes, relieving yourself into diapers. You long to be mothered and cared for extensively. (If you are lucky enough to find a partner who enjoys wiping smeared feces off of middle-aged men, everybody wins.)

Many Adult Babies are quite happy to spend their Friday nights goo-ing and gah-ing. For others, it can be a source of shame and can trigger bouts of depression.

CAUSALITY

Because so many Adult Babies are too busy having fun being Adult Babies to seek psychiatric treatment, very little research has gone into Adult Baby Syndrome. Some speculate it is caused by an emotional trauma that occurs in genuine infancy, while others assert that it stems from a subconscious desire to avoid the pressures and responsibilities of adult life.

> "You may enjoy wearing not only diapers but also baby's clothing in general."

Most Adult Babies do not want to be treated. And when one does, psychiatrists and psychologists are treading on little-worn terrain; treatment is usually administered on a case-by-case basis. Two methods that should probably be avoided are spanking and sending to the corner for time-outs, as these tend to encourage the disorder.

Of Note . . .

There are thousands, if not millions, of Internet sites that cater to Adult Babies' needs. Available for purchase are adult-sized diapers, adult-sized bibs, adult-sized jammies, all manner of adult-sized toys, and adult-sized prostitutes with a high tolerance for diaper-wearing weirdos.

KLÜVER–BUCY SYNDROME

Because sometimes you just want to lick stuff.

QUIZ YOURSELF

○ Do you ever forget important things?
○ Do you experience pleasure by exploring objects or people through touch?
○ Do you experience pleasure by exploring objects or people orally?
○ Do you ever experience periods of heightened sexual arousal?
○ Do you ever feel that your sex drive is more acute that most others'?

INNER MONOLOGUE

This dude has got to relax; he's taking this whole thing way too seriously. He acts like nobody ever licked his iPod before. Okay, hipster-man, everyone gets it; you're one of those technology freaks, and you're *too cool* to let strangers in doctors' waiting rooms examine your MP3 player with their tongues. Just ignore this jerk. Go sit across the room, let Captain Haircut enjoy his music in peace.

Hey, look, it's the new issue of *Yard & Garden*. What a

great magazine. Just feel those pages. So soft. So smooth. And an article called "How Sexy is Your Tractor?" That is a very, very sexy tractor. Those wheels, so big. And what an exhaust pipe! Oh, yeah. Oh, *Yard & Garden*.

Why is everybody staring at you? Haven't these people ever seen a man make love to a gardening magazine before? What a bunch of prudes.

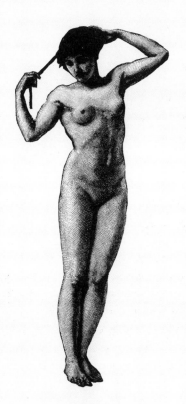

KLÜVER–BUCY
SYNDROME CONTINUED

DIAGNOSIS

Klüver-Bucy Syndrome is a fantastic disorder to have if you're looking for an excuse to grope perfect strangers and get your mouth all over their things, because when people get mad at you for what is widely considered to be inappropriate behavior, you can just say, "Hey, man, I've got Klüver-Bucy Syndrome. I can't help it." Then everyone laughs, and you can get back to sucking on the buttons of some guy's corduroy jacket.

While Klüver-Bucy Syndrome can cause a somewhat wide variety of odd symptoms—such as a deadening of emotions, bulimia, memory loss, and Prosopagnosia (see page 68)—those for which it's most commonly known are oral and tactile exploratory behavior (licking and feeling objects just because you want to) and hypersexuality (getting all freaky with people and objects just because you want to). While this kind of behavior may be perfectly acceptable at raves, in many other situations it can make people uncomfortable.

CAUSALITY

The disorder may be caused by lesions or damage to both the right and left medial temporal lobes of the brain, resulting from disease, injury, or epileptic seizure. Some doctors claim it could also occur after bilateral damage to the basolateral amygdala, but most hardcore basolateral amygdala enthusiasts aren't getting their hopes up without some solid evidence.

TREATMENT

Klüver-Bucy Syndrome, unfortunately, is untreatable. The symptoms, however, may be curbed independently, such as with antiandrogens, estrogens, and serotonergic drugs in the case of hypersexuality.

> ## Of Note . . .
>
> Klüver-Bucy Syndrome is named for Drs. Heinrich Klüver and Paul Bucy. In 1939, the two men bilaterally removed the temporal lobes of a group of rhesus monkeys, which then became hypersexual, masturbating and engaging in indiscriminate heterosexual and homosexual intercourse, following the surgery. Also named for the doctors is the Klüver-Bucy Maneuver, a sexual position in which a man has indiscriminate sex with a bisexual monkey.

PENIS PANIC
(ALSO KORO, GENITAL RETRACTION SYNDROME, SHOOK YANG, CASTRATION ANXIETY)

Because if there's one thing that will ruin your day, it's having your penis stolen.

QUIZ YOURSELF

- Does your penis vary in size throughout the course of the day?
- Do you find your penis to be significantly smaller now than it once was?
- Is your penis gone?
- Do you know of any sorcerers, witches, or foreigners who might like the opportunity to steal your penis?

INNER MONOLOGUE

Okay, no need to worry. You're in a crowded stadium. You're surrounded by football fans. That last time was a fluke. Just relax. Nobody is going to steal your penis.

But wait—what if one of these "football fans" is actually a wizard in disguise? Wizards are awfully good at disguising themselves. . . . Oh, you're being silly. Lightning doesn't strike twice. Well, at any rate, it doesn't strike four times. Just enjoy yourself and watch the game. There are so many people around, any wizard who might happen to be here could steal *anybody's* penis. Like that guy. He's good-looking; he probably has a very nice penis. He's the one who should be worrying. What an idiot, coming to a football game with that penis! Doesn't he know about the wizards?

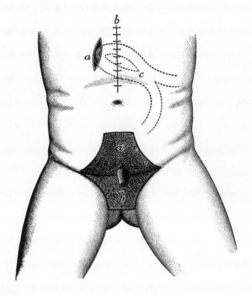

DIAGNOSIS

Penis Panic is not a metaphoric fear. It is not an aversion to feeling "unmanly," nor a fear of having to stop the car and ask for directions. It is the genuine belief that a wizard or witch or communist or criminal or terrorist is plotting to steal your penis or has stolen it already.

One would think it would be rather easy to verify whether your penis has been stolen. A quick trip to the men's room should do the trick, right? Wrong. A victim of Penis Panic suffers a sort of delusion, and despite efforts to prove to him that his penis is in his pants, where he always keeps it, he'll remain convinced that it is gone or is shrinking away.

Penis Panic can be infectious. Entire communities have been known to fall prey to mass hysteria, with people securing their penises with weights and clamps, wives and children holding onto the patriarchal member to keep it safe, and bands of vigilantes scouring the streets for the responsible party.

CAUSALITY

The male sexual organ has been known on occasion to become smaller than some men would like it to be. This can be caused by any number of things: illness, cold, anxiety, or even fear. So, if one man goes outside on a cold night and discovers that his penis isn't quite as glorious as it was when last he checked, he may jump to conclusions. And if that same man were to tell every other man he knows that a witch placed a hex on his penis and that it's shriveling to the size of a raisin, the fear that such a claim induces could actually cause other penises to shrink a bit. Two days later, an innocent woman is being chased through the streets, trying to avoid a lynching.

TREATMENT

Education about penises—how they work, how they expand and retract, how they are and are not affected by hexes, curses, and magical incantations—is the best means of calming and preventing Penis Panics.

> ## Of Note . . .
>
> In September 2003, a plague of "penis-melting robot combs" befell the men of the Sudanese capital of Khartoum. It was widely believed that the combs were a plot of West African Zionists intent on making all Sudanese men impotent. Panic was further spread when the rumors were corroborated by the local media. Of one incident, newspaper columnist Ja'far Abbas wrote, "No doubt, this comb was a laser-controlled surgical robot that penetrates the skull, passes to the lower body, and emasculates a man!!" Please go back and re-read that sentence.
>
> No actual evidence of penis melting was found by authorities.

SLEEP SEX
(ALSO SEXUAL BEHAVIOR IN SLEEP, SEXSOMNIA)

Because if this doesn't wake you up, nothing will.

QUIZ YOURSELF

○ Do you have little or no memory of the time you spent asleep last night?

○ Do you sometimes wake up feeling as though you didn't do anything horrible or damaging to your partner during the night?

○ Do you feel completely innocent of having forcibly engaged your partner in unwanted sexual activity?

INNER MONOLOGUE

What the—?! Why is your wife strangling you? And pushing her fingers into your eye socket? Seriously, not cool. There you were, sleeping peacefully on top of her, and she has to go and . . . wait a minute. Why were you sleeping on *top* of her? And why are your pajama bottoms bunched up around your ankles?

If you didn't know better, you might be led to believe you were in the middle of having sex. Except that your wife rarely strangles you or gouges your eyes during sex. Could it be that she doesn't want to be mounted at this hour? She's screaming. That's like sex. But this is a different kind of screaming—a decidedly less sexy kind. This is definitely a more scary kind of screaming.

This is bad. This is very, very bad. Maybe you should climb off your wife and apologize, and then try to figure out what the hell is going on.

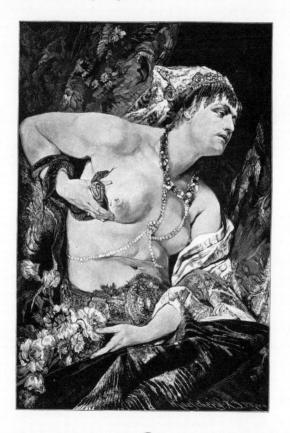

DIAGNOSIS

Sleep Sex is a relatively newly studied type of parasomnia, or sleep disorder, somewhat similar to sleepwalking, sleep talking, and Sleep Terror Disorder (page 188). People with Sleep Sex will engage in sexual activity while remaining fully asleep. This could mean masturbating yourself, masturbating whoever happens to be in bed with you, masturbating a roommate, masturbating a random person on the street outside your house, or having actual sex with just about anybody you stumble across. If you're lucky, this person will be a willing partner. If you're not lucky, you could be arrested.

Medical professionals are unclear on the disorder's exact nature; it's believed to be a form of REM (rapid eye movement) Behavioral Disorder. Normally, when a person enters the REM phase of sleep, he or she experiences muscle atonia, a sort of sleep paralysis that prevents the body from getting into trouble while dreaming. But with Sleep Sex, the paralysis is absent, meaning a person may physically enact his or her dreams. If these dreams happen to involve sex, which is not unlikely, the manifest symptoms of Sleep Sex can result.

If afflicted, you may become somewhat violent during Sleep Sex episodes—even if you tend to be perfectly gentle during waking sex. The good news is that you probably won't remember any of your activities in the morning. The bad news is that your partner almost certainly will.

CAUSALITY

Sleep Sex is most likely caused by the same brain arousal mechanism abnormalities that cause other parasomnias. It's thought to have a genetic component, but can be triggered by alcohol, drugs, stress, or severe exhaustion. Many people who experience Sleep Sex also suffer from other emotional and/or psychological problems, which is thought to be the difference between a sleepwalker and a sleepsexer.

TREATMENT

Drugs such as Valium and Klonopin have been known to help people with parasomnias regain muscle atonia and sleep peacefully through the night. However, any accompanying psychological or emotional problems should be dealt with as well. Psychotherapy may be recommended.

VAGINISMUS

Because you're not getting anything in there unless there wants it there.

○ Is sexual intercourse uncomfortable for you?
○ Is sexual intercourse extremely painful for you?
○ Is sexual intercourse simply impossible for you?

INNER MONOLOGUE

I'm sorry, but what exactly are you trying to squeeze in there? A penis? Alright, whose penis? And why exactly are you trying to get it in there? Sexual performance. I see. Well, let's take a look at the list. Hmmm . . . Penis, penis, penis . . . Sorry, but there doesn't appear to be a "penis" on the list. Nope, if it's not on the list, it's not getting through. It doesn't matter that you want the penis in there; you don't get to decide these things. What *is* on the list? Let's see. Hmmm . . . There doesn't appear to be anything on the list at this time. Sorry. The Vagina isn't taking visitors at this time.

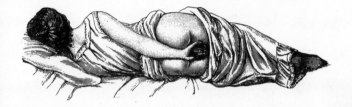

DIAGNOSIS

Although Vaginismus is a disorder that affects females, it can be one of the most frustrating things in the world for both women and men. Whenever one attempts to insert any object—be it penis, tampon, gynecological instrument, vibrator, dildo, carrot, Stretch Armstrong action figure—inside the vagina, the pubococcygeal muscle clamps shut. Access denied. You may not realize it, but those pubococcygeal muscles are quite strong.

Vaginismus is a reflex muscle reaction. It occurs without conscious decision and has nothing to do with your wishes, nor does it mean you are in any way averse to the insertion of an object. In fact, you might really, really want an object to be inserted.

In addition to being extremely annoying, it can also be very painful. Women have reported sharp pains when the pubococcygeal muscles clamp shut.

CAUSALITY

Vaginismus is caused by an innate, subconscious aversion to penetration. Somewhere in your brain, the idea of sex equates to "wrong." This can be due to apprehension about sexual intimacy, religious beliefs, or a past sexual trauma. These are things that do not come immediately to mind; they can be deeply repressed. Often, you will have no idea why this is occurring, and may simply wish it would stop.

A vaginal infection or childbirth can also lead to the disorder, as can experiencing a painful sexual encounter immediately following such a situation.

"Vaginismus occurs without conscious decision and has nothing to do with your wishes."

Vaginismus is usually cured through two steps: psychological therapy—to help the patient figure out and understand *why* this is happening, so that the problem can be dealt with—and physical therapy, in which a series of dilators of increasing size are inserted into the vagina over the course of several months, allowing the muscles to slowly acclimate to the sensation of foreign objects.

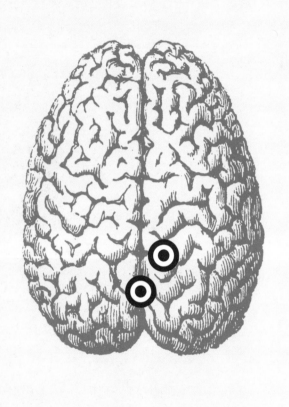

SLEEP
DISORDERS

Because sleep is the deep, black void
we must each enter every night.

HMONG SUDDEN DEATH SYNDROME

(ALSO SUDDEN UNEXPECTED NOCTURNAL DEATH SYNDROME, VOODOO DEATH, BANGUNGUT)

Because sometimes death will come as a demonic female spirit in the night.

QUIZ YOURSELF

○ Do you feel healthy?
○ Is everything pretty much normal with you, physically?
○ Do you have no history of sleep disorders?
○ Have you died for no good reason while sleeping?

INNER MONOLOGUE

Damn it! You never called your parents for their anniversary, you idiot! They get so sensitive about that kind of thing, especially your mom. She won't let you forget that. What time is it? Ten o'clock? Oh, they've long since gone to bed. You're just going to have to remember to call them in the morning. Well, unless you die for no good reason in the middle of the night. But otherwise, you'll have to call them in the morning.

Oh, and assuming you don't die for no good reason in

the middle of the night, you also have to remember to buy cat food.

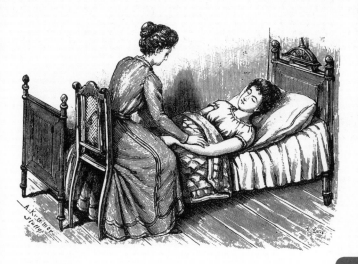

DIAGNOSIS

What happens with Hmong Sudden Death Syndrome is that one night you kiss your wife goodnight and lie down comfortably in your bed for a restful night's sleep, and then, while you're sleeping, you just die for no good reason. Okay, not for *no* good reason; the cause of death is technically a sudden heart attack, but the heart attack isn't linked to any physical origin. You experience something resembling a major panic attack while completely asleep, and this induces a heart attack, and the heart attack induces your death. The whole thing is over before you know it's happening.

CAUSALITY

Hmong Sudden Death Syndrome occurs most frequently in men—from Laos or the Philippines—in their mid-thirties who have recently moved away from their homes. Many times, they are former soldiers who have suffered trauma prior to relocating. More than 100 such cases have been reported in the U.S. alone since the Centers for Disease Control and Prevention started collecting data in 1981.

The syndrome is thought to be triggered by the combination of stress and guilt at having left a tumultuous former life behind, difficulty readjusting to life in a new country, and a cultural belief in nocturnal visits from an evil female spirit who likes to suffocate people in their sleep.

To date, there is no medical explanation for why this syndrome should occur, particularly in such a small, culturally specific set of people. But doctors continue to investigate, studying the effects of sleep apnea, heart disease genetics, and nutrition, among other factors. Even so, the importance of the evil female spirit who likes to suffocate people while they sleep should not be discounted.

"To date, there is no medical explanation for why this syndrome should occur."

Not really an option, for obvious reasons.

Of Note . . .

One former Laotian who did manage to survive Hmong Sudden Death Syndrome describes three increasingly difficult nights he experienced shortly after moving to the United States: On the first night, he awoke and saw a cat sitting on his chest. On the next night, he watched a dark figure, something like a strange-looking dog, walk to his bed and climb onto his chest, making it difficult for him to breathe. On the third night, he lay unmoving in horror as a tall, pale-skinned female spirit floated into his room, pinned him to his bed, and kept him from breathing with her weight. He woke up screaming, and the next day he sought help from a shaman who relieved him of a collective of unhappy spirits. From that day forward, he slept fine.

SLEEP TERROR DISORDER
(ALSO PAVOR NOCTURNUS, NIGHT TERROR)

Because we all have to face our demons.

QUIZ YOURSELF

○ Do you scream at the top of your lungs in the middle of the night?

○ Do people not want to fall asleep near you?

INNER MONOLOGUE

Whoa, it's getting late. You can barely keep your eyes open. Maybe you should check and see what's on C-SPAN. Oh, look, it's a guy talking about a book about stock portfolios. You always wanted to know about state tax analysis.

No, no, come on, this is ridiculous. You don't care about state tax analysis. You have to go to bed. Your body needs sleep. And it probably won't happen tonight. Probably. You probably won't wake up screaming with the feeling that all is bad in the world, that a nameless, faceless, malevolent dread is pushing weightily down upon your chest. You probably won't startle yourself awake, crying, panicked, in a pool of your own sweat. And you probably won't come to understand all too well how, in certain miserable mind-states, even death seems like a welcomed, merciful release from the sepulchre of utter despair.

On second thought, state tax analysis really would be a good thing to understand.

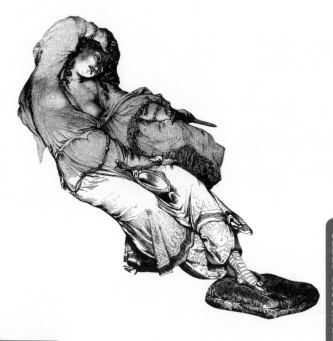

DIAGNOSIS

The effects of Sleep Terror Disorder are no ordinary, run-of-the-mill bad dreams. Unlike nightmares—which generally occur during the lighter sleep stages, those closer to the point of natural waking—"Night Terrors" take place during periods of very deep, non-REM sleep. Because of this, they are rarely associated with images or narratives, so there's nothing specific to pin the fear onto. Instead, Sleep Terror manifests itself as the pure, intensely felt emotion of fear or dread.

As a Sleep Terror sufferer, you will commonly wake up screaming, gasping for air, or moaning the moan of a person who has gazed into the eye sockets of death. You will feel disoriented, bogged down with an intangible sense of horror. This is sometimes accompanied by a short period of amnesia and possibly paralysis. Within ten to twenty minutes, the ordeal should end on its own, but not without leaving its psychological, and often physical, mark. Victims may suffer from depression, lack of concentration, fatigue, stomach problems, muscle aches, and headaches as secondary effects.

CAUSALITY

The exact cause of Sleep Terror Disorder is uncertain, but several centuries ago, it was believed that uneasy sleep was caused by a demon sitting on the victim's chest. This is almost certainly not true. More likely causes include emotional stress, internal conflict, and gloom faeries.

"You will commonly wake up moaning the moan of a person who has gazed into the eye sockets of death."

In many cases, Sleep Terror Disorder will simply go away after a few weeks, when its causes cease or go back into the forest. If episodes persist, counseling, psychotherapy, or hypnosis may be recommended. In some cases, sleep medications such as diazepam may be prescribed.

SLEEP DISORDERS

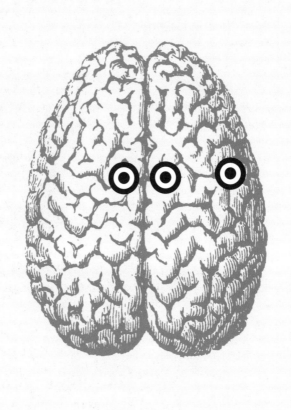

SOMATOFORM DISORDERS

*Because what we perceive
is not always what's perceivable.*

BODY DYSMORPHIC DISORDER
(ALSO DISMORPHOPHOBIA)

Because it's cruel to subject the world to the horrifying image of that slight bump on your nose, which you can totally almost see if you look really, really closely with a magnifying glass.

QUIZ YOURSELF

○ Are you sensitive about your appearance?

○ Are there things about the way you look that you would like to change?

○ Do you worry that people judge you as unattractive?

○ Do you bear any unsightly physical features that glow as beacons of proof that God does not love His children?

INNER MONOLOGUE

You can do this. Just walk out the door, go around the corner, and buy a pack of coffee filters. You're being way too sensitive. Nobody on the street is going to stare at you, pointing in horror. Nobody is going to squeal and gawk at the quarter-inch scar on your left cheek. Nobody's going to think, *"Holy Mother of God!* What *terrible* misfortune did that young lady suffer to make her so hideously grotesque? Did she somehow survive a fall into a wheat thresher?!"

Will they?

No . . . No, that's not going to happen. This is all in your head. Now, take your horrible disgusting deformity and go buy some coffee filters.

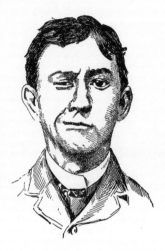

DIAGNOSIS

Body Dysmorphic Disorder has nothing to do with being genuinely unattractive or having a real physical defect. In fact, there are probably a number of less-than-attractive people who could benefit from a touch of Body Dysmorphic Disorder. (Weird-looking lumpy guy who insists on walking around the locker room without a towel, please take note.) But people with this disorder, despite looking perfectly normal or even quite beautiful, will feel certain that they are simply too ugly for visual consumption. They may exaggerate the size of their nose, the prominence of scars or acne, the density of facial hair, or the asymmetry of their face or body. Or, they may simply imagine a problem where none exists at all.

If you suffer from Body Dysmorphic Disorder, your defects will seem very real, and the ruminations on them will be all-encompassing. You may spend hours each day staring unhappily at your reflection. You may avoid going outside. You may quit your job so that your coworkers don't have to endure your ugliness. You may do what you can to hide your "problem" using makeup or clothing or veils, but nothing will really help, because the problem is not physically there.

CAUSALITY

Body Dysmorphic Disorder affects men and women at about the same rate, approximately 2 percent of the population, and usually begins in the teens or early 20s, while most people are still formulating a physical self-image. It tends to affect perfectionists, people with overly rigid personal goals. For these people, nothing about themselves can equal their own expectations, and in the case of this disorder, this self-esteem problem manifests itself physically.

Some doctors believe that many with Body Dysmorphic Disorder are biologically predisposed toward a mental disorder, and that it may be caused by an imbalance of serotonin within the brain. If this is the case, then it may be triggered by use of serotonin-releasing drugs, such as methylenedioxymethamphetamine (known as ecstasy).

TREATMENT

Most cases of Body Dysmorphic Disorder go untreated, because people with the disorder don't believe they have one. When they look in the mirror, they see ugliness, and can't understand why others don't as well.

When treatment is sought, cognitive behavioral therapy, in which a psychologist teaches the patient to avoid obsessing on his or her physical appearance, or anti-obsessional medication—antidepressants that affect serotonin levels, such as Prozac—may be prescribed.

Of Note...

Many people with Body Dysmorphic Disorder will seek plastic surgery instead of therapy. This rarely improves how they view their physical appearance, and often makes them feel worse, not to mention a couple thousand dollars poorer.

BODY INTEGRITY IDENTITY DISORDER

Because sometimes two legs is 0.7563 legs too many.

QUIZ YOURSELF

- O Do you ever have feelings of incompleteness?
- O Do you ever feel depressed, or alone in the world?
- O Do you suffer pangs of envy while staring wistfully at amputees?
- O Do you experience fantasies of life after amputation?
- O Have you ever purposefully mutilated one of your limbs in the hopes of having it removed surgically?

INNER MONOLOGUE

You should be proud of yourself—you have it all. A happy marriage, loving children, a five-figure job with benefits including dental, an eye-care plan, even a company car. You're living the American dream. What could be wrong? What's this feeling of incompleteness that follows you through each new success? Why can't you shake it?

Oh, you know the reason. Just thinking of it now sends thrills down your spine, little waves of electric excitement that flicker down at your thigh—precisely the locus of your unhappiness. In your fantasies, you've already taken action.

With the clever use of a belt and a pair of pinned-up pants, you've been simulating it for years. *Hours* spent staring at your reflection—your artificially corrected self—in the mirrored closet door. In those hours, you're happy. In that imaginary time, you're complete.

Truth is, that left leg simply has to go. And if you can't find a doctor to perform the surgery, you're going to have to do it yourself. Not the whole leg, no. But from the spot 15/19ths of an inch above the kneecap on down to your foot—none of it can stay. You should never have been born with those insufferable inches. Really, what kind of a vengeful god would curse you with such an obviously *not*-missing leg?

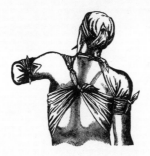

DIAGNOSIS

Body Integrity Identity Disorder, the desire to have one or more body parts amputated, is not a form of psychosis. There is no bending of reality or impaired judgment involved. In fact, if you are diagnosed with

Psychosis, you cannot technically have Body Integrity Identity Disorder. People with the disorder genuinely want to have an arm or leg or what-have-you lopped off.

And not just any arm or leg or what-have-you. If you suffer from the disorder, you will know exactly which limb and, often, the exact point at which the limb needs to go. Every day with the offending limb still attached is a troubled day. You will covet the not-limb of amputees, and you may even hide an arm beneath a shirt or tuck a leg up in your pants and go out into the world as though you were one.

CAUSALITY

There are no known reasons for Body Integrity Identity Disorder. Many victims begin to desire amputation during early childhood, usually after seeing, and feeling jealousy toward, an amputee. Without fully understanding it, they will form a sensation of incompleteness that will find its locus at the limb that shouldn't be there. In this sense, it is similar to Gender Identity Disorder, in which men harbor a desire to be women and women harbor a desire to be men and 30 percent of both harbor a desire to discuss their desires on trashy talk shows.

The best known treatment for wanting to have your arm cut off is to have your arm cut off. Usually, a post-operative patient will feel satisfied with the decision and go on with his or her life, minus the unwanted portion. Some hospitals are sympathetic to the condition and will admit patients with Body Integrity Identity Disorder, but these facilities are rare. Absent willing medical help, some sufferers will intentionally mangle or destroy the limb to necessitate amputation. Others will simply perform the task themselves, by whatever means available.

Of Note . . .

Body Integrity Identity Disorder is not to be confused with Acrotomophilia, which is a sexual attraction to other people who are missing limbs. But if you happen to know one person with one disorder and another with the other one, and you haven't yet introduced them . . .

DELUSIONS OF PARASITOSIS

(ALSO EKBOM SYNDROME, MONOSYMPOMATIC
HYPOCHONDRIASIS, DERMATOZOENWAHN)

*Because believing you are infested with thousands of worms can be worse
than actually being infested with thousands of worms.*

QUIZ YOURSELF

○ Are you certain that bugs and worms are oozing from
   your pores?
○ Do friends claim to not see bugs and worms oozing from
   your pores?
○ Do doctors claim to not find any evidence that bugs and
   worms are oozing from your pores?
○ Why is everybody lying to you?

INNER MONOLOGUE

You should never have agreed to come on this date. Not until
you've taken care of your . . . problem. A fancy restaurant
like this is no place for you; you're infested with worms. You
can feel them right now, squirming beneath the fabric of
this dress you couldn't really afford. Try not to show your
revulsion. Don't let him catch on.

He is handsome, though, isn't he? And so kind. Maybe he'll understand. Maybe you should explain that it's not your fault but somehow tiny little worms got inside your body and started to breed and now they're everywhere. . . . No, of course he won't understand! Why should he? It's disgusting. You're disgusting. You're a virtual worm hotel.

God, he's looking deeply into your eyes. You're starting to sweat. Please don't let a dozen or so worms come crawling out of your cheeks now. He'll throw up all over your dress, and then you won't be able to take it back to the store. You can't take it back anyway; it's filled with worms. Ugh, they're all over you. Squirming. In your bra, your underwear. You can feel a clump of them bunched up beneath your panty-hose by your ankle. You have to leave. Leave now. It's only a matter of time before he notices. Get out. Go!

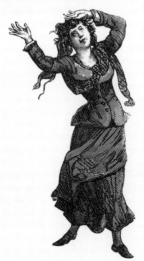

DELUSIONS OF PARASITOSIS CONTINUED

DIAGNOSIS

Parasitosis is the condition of being infested with parasites, such as mites, lice, worms, or maggots. *Delusions* are strongly held beliefs that persist despite a lack of evidence. *Of* is a preposition, used to show the relation between two nouns. When placed together like this: "of Parasitosis Delusions," they are a bunch of nonsense. However, when placed in another order, they can be a terrifying mental disorder.

If you suffer from Delusions of Parasitosis, you will believe your body is teeming with bugs. You can feel them crawling beneath your skin, you can see them emerging from your pores and orifices, you will find them floating in the toilet after relieving yourself. It's a nightmare. One might think it's better to *think* you're infested with maggots than to actually *be* infested with maggots, but consider this: You can have actual maggots extracted from your body. How do you get rid of imaginary maggots?

CAUSALITY

Delusions of Parasitosis can be triggered by actual diseases—such as diabetes, tuberculosis, or syphilis—that affect multiple organs and perceptual mechanisms. The syndrome is also a well-known aspect of Delirium Tremens, a complication of serious alcohol withdrawal. In some cases, however, the delusions are preceded by an *actual* parasite infestation. You get some maggots crawling around beneath your skin once and it can be pretty hard to shake that feeling.

TREATMENT

Many cases go untreated. Dermatologists are not usually equipped to deal with psychiatric problems, so the best they can do is assure the patient there are no bugs. And most people with Delusions of Parasitosis do not want to be directed to a psychiatrist, because they don't want to be analyzed; they want to be fumigated.

In some cases, a dermatologist will prescribe anti-parasite medicine as though the patient were actually infested. Sometimes this will help satisfy the mind, but because the stem problem is often a slight psychosis, placebo medication doesn't always work. A growing belief is that the dermatologist should encourage the patient to seek psychological help, not for the delusions per se, but for the feelings of depression or shame that may accompany parasitic infestation. From there, a psychiatrist can treat the problem properly.

SOMATOFORM DISORDERS

APPENDIX A: Phobias

A phobia is an irrational fear of a specific object or situation, marked by severe anxiety sometimes culminating in a full-blown panic attack. Often, a phobia can be incredibly debilitating, keeping its victim from performing everyday tasks. Phobias are usually treated with cognitive behavioral therapy, and sometimes drugs, such as antidepressants, anti-anxiety medications, and beta blockers, may be prescribed.

The following is a far-from-complete list of some known phobias:

Ablutophobia: fear of bathing
Ambulophobia: fear of walking
Anablephobia: fear of looking up
Anthrophobia: fear of flowers
Asymmetriphobia: fear of asymmetry
Atomosophobia: fear of atomic explosions
Aulophobia: fear of flutes
Barophobia: fear of gravity
Bibliophobia: fear of books
Bolshephobia: fear of Bolsheviks
Carnophobia: fear of meat
Cathisophobia: fear of sitting
Catoptrophobia: fear of mirrors
Chaetophobia: fear of hair
Chirophobia: fear of hands
Chronomentrophobia: fear of clocks
Coulrophobia: fear of clowns
Cyclophobia: fear of bicycles
Defecaloesiophobia: fear of painful bowel movements
Domatophobia: fear of houses
Eleutherophobia: fear of freedom
Ephebiphobia: fear of teenagers
Euphobia: fear of hearing good news
Geliophobia: fear of laughter
Gymnophobia: fear of nudity
Hagiophobia: fear of holy things
Heliophobia: fear of the sun
Hippopotomonstrosesquippedaliophobia: fear of long words
Hobophobia: fear of beggars
Ichthyophobia: fear of fish
Kleptophobia: fear of stealing
Lachanophobia: fear of vegetables
Leukophobia: fear of the color white
Levophobia: fear of things to the left side of the body
Liticaphobia: fear of lawsuits

Lutraphobia: fear of otters
Macrophobia: fear of long waits
Medorthophobia: fear of an erect penis
Metrophobia: fear of poetry
Microbiophobia: fear of microbes
Novercaphobia: fear of stepmothers
Octophobia: fear of the figure "8"
Oenophobia: fear of wines
Ommatophobia: fear of eyes
Oneirogmophobia: fear of wet dreams
Orthophobia: fear of property
Panophobia: fear of everything
Papyrophobia: fear of paper
Parthenophobia: fear of virgins
Pediophobia: fear of dolls
Peladophobia: fear of bald people
Phobophobia: fear of phobias
Phronemophobia: fear of thinking
Podophobia: fear of feet
Proctophobia: fear of rectums
Pteronophobia: fear of being tickled by feathers
Pupaphobia: fear of puppets
Scopophobia: fear of being stared at
Somniphobia: fear of sleep
Spacephobia: fear of outer space
Syngenesophobia: fear of relatives
Theatrophobia: fear of theatres
Tremophobia: fear of trembling
Tyrannophobia: fear of tyrants
Uranophobia: fear of heaven
Venustraphobia: fear of beautiful women
Verbophobia: fear of words
Xenoglossophobia: fear of foreign languages
Xylophobia: fear of wooden objects
Zemmiphobia: fear of the great mole rat

APPENDIX B: Manias

A mania is an obsessive preoccupation with a specific object, concept, or action. To the victim, his or her mania is all-encompassing, refusing to be ignored until attention has been paid. Attempts to ignore the mania may lead to extreme anxiety. Most manias can be treated through behavior modification therapy, and sometimes with prescription drugs, such as antidepressants.

The following are just a few examples of documented manias:

Ablutomania: obsessive desire to bathe

Acronymania: obsession with acronyms

Ailuromania: intense enthusiasm for cats

Apimania: obsession with bees

Arithmomania: obsessive preoccupation with counting

Cacodemonomania: obsessive belief that one is possessed by an evil spirit

Cacospectamania: obsession with staring at repulsive things

Catapedamania: obsession with jumping from high places

Chinamania: obsession with collecting china

Chionomania: obsessive desire for snow

Cingulomania: overwhelming urge to hold a woman in one's arms

Clinomania: excessive desire to stay in bed

Chiromania: obsessive compulsion to masturbate

Coprolalomania: obsession with foul language

Copromania: obsession with feces

Discomania: obsession for disco music

Doromania: abnormal desire to give presents

Ecdemomania: compulsion to wander

Edeomania: obsession with genitals

Empleomania: obsession with holding public office

Epomania: craze for writing epic poems

Eulogomania: obsessive fondness for eulogies

Gamomania: overwhelming urge to make marriage proposals

Glazomania: obsessive list-making

Gynonudomania: overwhelming urge to rip off a woman's clothes

Hippomania: obsession with horses

Infomania: excessive devotion to accumulating facts

Islomania: obsession with islands

Klazomania: compulsion to shout

Mentulomania: obsession with the penis

Misomania: obsessive hatred of all things

Netomania: addiction to the Internet

Oniomania: uncontrollable urge to buy things

Onychotillomania: compulsion to mutilate one's fingernails and toenails

Orchidomania: obsession with orchids

Plutomania: obsession with money

Politicomania: obsession with politics

Polkamania: obsession with polka dancing

Poriomania: compulsion to aimlessly wander

Pseudomania: irrational predilection for lying

Rhinotillexomania: compulsive nose-picking

Rinkomania: obsession with skating

Siderodromomania: obsession with railroad travel

Trichomania: obsession with hair

Triskaidekamania: obsession with the number thirteen

Turkomania: obsession with all things Turkish

Typomania: obsession with having one's writing published

Xenomania: obsessive interest in foreigners

ACKNOWLEDGMENTS

There are so many people I would like to thank that the list itself could be published under a separate cover as *The Obsessive-Compulsive Author's Pocket Guide to People I'd Like to Acknowledge Here in the Acknowledgments*. However, I've been advised that that book probably wouldn't sell very well. So, here, unfortunately, is an extremely abridged version:

. . . Susan DiClaudio, Dennis DiClaudio, Sr., Denelle DiClaudio, Anthony DiClaudio, Diandra DiClaudio, Carmen Panarello, Anthony DiMaggio, Ray DiClaudio, and my entire family . . .

. . . Amy Wideman, Kate Perry, and all the fine folks at becker&mayer! . . .

. . . Yelena Gitlin, Colin Dickerman, Panio Gianopoulos, Benjamin Adams, and everyone at Bloomsbury USA . . .

. . . Paula Balzer . . .

. . . and every one of my friends, all of whom have requested not to be "outed" as such in such a public fashion. I totally, totally understand.

Thank you all so much!